GAY MEN'S HEALTH

A Guide to the AID Syndrome and Other Sexually Transmitted Diseases

GAY MEN'S HEALTH

A Guide to the AID Syndrome and Other Sexually Transmitted Diseases

JEANNE KASSLER, M.D.

1817

HARPER & ROW, PUBLISHERS, New York
Cambridge, Philadelphia, San Francisco.
London, Mexico City, São Paulo, Sydney

To R.K. and F.K.

 For information address Harper & Row, Publishers, Inc., 10 East 53rd Street, New York, N.Y. 10022. Published simultaneously in Canada by Fitzhenry & Whiteside Limited, Toronto.

FIRST EDITION

Library of Congress Cataloging in Publication Data

Kassler, Jeanne.
Gay men's health.

Bibliography: p.
Includes index.
1. Venereal diseases. 2. Homosexuals, Male—Diseases. 3. Acquired immune deficiency syndrome. I. Title.
RC200.2.K37 1983 616.95'1 82–48669
ISBN 0–06–015146–3 83 84 85 86 87 88 10 9 8 7 6 5 4 3 2 1
ISBN 0–06–091057–7 (pbk.) 83 84 85 86 87 88 10 9 8 7 6 5 4 3 2 1

CONTENTS

ACKNOWLEDGMENTS

I would like to thank the people who took time from their busy schedules to be interviewed: Mark Behar, Larry Kramer, and doctors Hardy Kornfeld, Paul Paroski, Bijan Safai, Peter Seitzman, David Sencer, Barbara Starrett, and Daniel William. A particular thanks goes to Dr. William for reading the final manuscript.

I would also like to thank the staff of the St. Mark's Clinic, all of whom volunteer their labor to promote the health of their patients.

The Centers for Disease Control deserves special mention for their prompt cooperation in sending me valuable publications, which served as a foundation for much of this book.

I would especially like to thank Carol Cohen, my editor at Harper & Row, for her invaluable help in preparing the manuscript and for the warmth and tact with which her suggestions were made. Special thanks go to Nancy Trichter, agent and friend, for helping turn this project into a reality, and also to Dr. Donald Gemson, who often provided a "second opinion."

Louis Slesin deserves thanks for closely watching developments that affect the health of many, and for bringing relevant information to my attention. And I would like to thank Barbara Fried and Patricia O'Brien simply for intelligent friendship, which in the end is far from simple.

It is also fair to say that without the technology of my Sanyo micro-computer, this book might not exist.

Jeanne Kassler

March 1983

INTRODUCTION

During the 1950s it must have seemed that penicillin would usher in an era of VD control. But the statistics of the 1980s show otherwise. The incidence of gonorrhea has tripled since the 1960s and syphilis is on the rise. Even the diseases that penicillin can cure have not been eradicated.

Fifteen years ago there were five infections that were recognized as sexually transmitted diseases. Now there are more than twenty. Syphilis, gonorrhea, granuloma inguinale, chancroid, and lymphogranuloma venereum are still with us, but today's list is much longer and includes many infections for which there are no easy cures.

Sexually transmitted diseases (STDs) are a national epidemic. Although they are a worldwide problem, infection rates are considerably higher in the United States than in many other Western countries.

"STD" may be an unfamiliar term but it isn't linguistic vogue that has caused "venereal disease" and its acronym "VD" to be replaced by "sexually transmitted diseases" and "STD." STD is an umbrella term that includes a broader range of infections than was ever suggested by the term VD.

The switch occurred because only the mode of transmission—and not the symptoms—link many STDs to sex. "Sexually transmitted diseases" often forsake the apparent connection between cause (i.e. sex) and effect (i.e. genital sores) that is implied by "venereal diseases." The symptoms may be unrelated to the sexual organs; for example, hepatitis—now a major STD—doesn't cause genital symptoms.

Many STDs can also be transmitted nonsexually; hepatitis B can be passed on through blood transfusions. But once sexual transmission explains why many people have a disease, the infection joins the roster of STDs.

What has caused this epidemic of STDs?

The sexual revolution is usually blamed. The argument is that today's plight is the predictable outcome of lots of people having lots of partners, especially when they don't use condoms or spermicidal creams, which help prevent disease transmission. Although there is truth in this argument, the change in sexual habits, by itself, doesn't explain the current problem. There are multiple reasons.

People usually know very little about sexually transmitted diseases. Unfortunately, the liberalization of attitudes toward sex hasn't been followed by a liberalization of attitudes toward STDs. As a result, many people still only learn about them "through the fragmentary lessons of disease acquisition."*

This is partly due to the medical profession's neglect of STDs. A 1980 government report stated that "the current STD epidemic is rooted in ignorance, apathy, and neglect. Nowhere are this apathy and neglect more apparent than in the medical profession itself."† A 1982 study found that only 30 percent of American medical students receive any training in venereology—and they get an average of six hours of instruction.

The neglect is reflected in the lack of funds available for STD research, training, and treatment. In 1980, only $90 million of the total $54-billion health-care budget was earmarked for STD control. And yet the financial consequences of STDs are enormous. Gonorrhea alone was said to have cost $770 million in 1978.

The split between private and public medical care compounds the problem. Many private physicians don't have the time to track down sexual contacts of patients with STDs to ensure that their partners are also treated. Yet contact tracing is a vital aspect of STD control. While public-health officials will trace contacts for private practitioners, a 1977 report from New York City showed that more than 40 percent of doctors refused to allow public-health authorities to approach their patients, citing issues of confidentiality.

Patients are often reluctant to seek treatment, because they are embarrassed, don't know where to go, or fear the financial consequences. If they go to local public-health clinics, they may find drab and poorly staffed facilities. And poorly funded clinics do not inspire

* Robert K. Bolan, "Sexually Transmitted Diseases in Homosexuals: Focusing the Attack," *Sexually Transmitted Diseases* (1981) 8:296.

† National Institutes of Allergy and Infectious Diseases, *Sexually Transmitted Diseases, 1980 Status Report* NIAID Study Group, NIH publication no. 81-2213, p. 10.

patients to return for further, necessary care.

While STDs are a potential problem for everyone who isn't celibate, gay men and heterosexual women suffer the most. Although this book discusses only the problem that STDs pose for gay men, let it be said that STDs inflict untold numbers of forced sterilizations and ectopic pregnancies on women and debilitating infections on their offspring.

But how are STDs special for gay men?

First, the actual diseases can be different. Certain infections, such as amebiasis and giardiasis, are not often seen in the straight community although they are common STDs among gay men. The reason is that some infections are transmitted through oral-anal sex and anal-receptive intercourse. Were these sexual practices more widespread in the straight community, there is no medical reason why many of the STDs now seen almost exclusively in the gay community wouldn't become more prevalent among heterosexuals. It is the sexual practices rather than the gender of one's partners that are responsible.

The traditional venereal diseases may also cause different symptoms among gay men than they do among straight men because the site of infection isn't the same. Syphilis and gonorrhea are common rectal infections in gay men, whereas they tend to be genital infections in straight men. Old diseases can have new places.

But it isn't only that the diseases may be different; a higher proportion of gay men than straight men seem to suffer from STDs. This sets up a vicious cycle within the community. As more people become infected, it gets progressively easier to catch an STD from each new partner. It is much easier to catch something if 5 out of 10 people have it than if only 1 out of 10 has it.

Many people have infections that cause no symptoms and therefore go untreated, but they remain contagious and cause the community's infection rate to increase. Anonymous sexual partners make the situation more difficult because contact tracing becomes impossible. The high rates of infection are self-perpetuating.

Finally, gay men today face the special threat of AID syndrome, or AIDS, the life-threatening acquired immune deficiency syndrome that came to light in 1981. Although AIDS is not restricted to gay men, 72 percent of cases do occur in gay men. And AIDS seems to be a sexually transmitted disease. While acquiring an infection that can be easily cured may be inconvenient, the risk of acquiring a deadly disease makes prevention imperative. AIDS has raised the ante of STDs, removing the sense of security that antibiotics once provided.

The pages that follow describe the STDs that affect gay men—what they are, their symptoms, what sexual practices are most likely to transmit them, how they are diagnosed and treated, and what can be done to prevent them. Although each disease is described individually, in reality people often have more than one STD at a time. The treatment recommendations are usually those suggested by the Centers for Disease Control in their latest 1982 bulletin.

Education provides protection against having to learn by unwanted experience. It permits one to make decisions that are genuinely based on informed consent.

The sexually transmitted diseases are described in this book for informational purposes only. If the reader believes he is suffering from any of these diseases, he should seek professional medical advice.

THE ACQUIRED IMMUNE DEFICIENCY SYNDROME (AIDS)

On June 5, 1981, the Centers for Disease Control (CDC) first alerted the medical community that five previously healthy, gay men from Los Angeles had developed *Pneumocystis carinii* pneumonia (PCP), a rare infection that was not known to occur in persons with healthy immune systems.

Four weeks later, on July 3, the Centers for Disease Control reported that Kaposi's sarcoma (KS), a cancer not known to strike healthy young Americans, had been found in 26 gay men from New York and California during the previous 30 months. An update on the problem of *Pneumocystis carinii* pneumonia revealed that an additional 10 cases among gay men had been reported in the intervening month and that unusual cases of herpes simplex were also being seen.

While PCP and KS were known to afflict patients whose immune systems were impaired, either by disease or by medical treatment of serious disorders, there was no known explanation for the immune suppression in these gay men.

The acquired immune deficiency syndrome, better known as AIDS, was a new problem whose fundamental feature was a malfunctioning immune system, recognized because of the appearance of rare infections and cancers. PCP and KS were not the new diseases; the predisposition to this rare infection and cancer was new. An unknown cause was destroying the immune defenses of previously healthy young homosexual men.

That new diseases appear periodically was not the surprise. Legionnaires' pneumonia was first recognized during a 1976 outbreak in Philadelphia that killed 34 of its 221 victims. Four years later, toxic shock syndrome, a disease that primarily affects young menstruating women, erupted as a new medical problem; it killed 84 of its 1,600 victims. And both of these diseases still occur.

But although these outbreaks gripped the public imagination at the time, they pall in the light of today's new epidemic. Numerically, they were less significant. AIDS has already killed more people than Legionnaires' disease and toxic shock syndrome combined. And while the number of persons afflicted with AIDS is sufficient to make it a national public-health concern, the numbers alone don't explain the medical significance of AIDS, nor the fear that it has engendered.

AIDS is the first known naturally occurring breakdown of the body's immune system, a system that is the body's basic defense against the continuous onslaught of infectious agents and malignant transformations of the body's own cells. Without a working immune system, no one survives for any length of time.

Unlike previous infectious diseases, such as Legionnaires' pneumonia, the vast majority of AIDS patients who survive the initial illness don't really recover. Instead, they go on to develop other diseases because the underlying defect—a faulty immune system—seems virtually incapable of correction once it has been severely damaged. Thirty-six percent of AIDS patients have already died, and many investigators fear that the death rate will go much higher because the surviving patients fail to regain normal immune function. Seventy-five percent of those patients who were diagnosed before 1982 have already died.

In June 1981, the CDC formed an AIDS task force of more than 100 investigators, but, two years later, no one yet knows what causes AIDS. However, the epidemiology of AIDS—the study of who gets it—now suggests that AIDS is probably an infectious disease.

Roughly 72 percent of AIDS patients are gay men who live in large urban centers. Forty-five percent of AIDS patients live in New York City, 12 percent in San Francisco, 6 percent in Los Angeles. Miami, Newark, and Houston are also reporting significant numbers of cases. The clustering of AIDS in a particular group and in certain geographic locations was the first clue that AIDS had an environmental cause—either an infectious agent or some other aspect of a shared "life-style."

But while gay men accounted for all the first reported cases, new groups have been steadily added to the list. Heterosexual men and women who use intravenous drugs now account for 17 percent of AIDS cases. On July 9, 1982, the CDC reported that 34 Haitians—

none of whom was gay and only one of whom used intravenous drugs—became the third group of people to get AIDS; they account for 5 percent of cases. Then, on July 16, 1982, a fourth group was added: patients with hemophilia A, a bleeding disorder that requires frequent administration of blood products to replace missing clotting factors; they account for 0.9 percent of cases.

The remaining 6 percent of AIDS patients didn't fit any of these classifications. Some were the children and sexual partners of intravenous-drug users; some were children and elderly adults who had received blood transfusions. In December 1982 a 20-month-old infant became the youngest patient to die of AIDS.

Not only were more types of people falling prey to AIDS but the number of people with AIDS was rising at an alarming rate. The CDC estimated that there were twice as many cases every six months. Looking at past hospital records, the CDC found three cases of AIDS prior to 1978. In January 1981 there was approximately one new case a day. By March 1983, the CDC was being notified of four to five new cases a day, and the total number of cases was 1240. AIDS had been reported in 34 states and 15 foreign countries, including Germany, France, and Denmark.

Despite the diversity of people who got AIDS, there was a common thread. The link was that hepatitis B was also prevalent in those groups at greatest risk for AIDS: gay men, intravenous drug users, and patients who receive blood transfusions or blood derivatives. Both hepatitis B, which is caused by a virus, and AIDS were probably transmitted in the same ways: by sexual contact, contaminated needles, and blood transfusions. And both diseases were likely to have a similar cause: a virus.

It isn't entirely clear how the Haitians fit into the picture. The current feeling is that if AIDS is caused by a virus, the virus may have originated in Haiti. The recent finding of 11 cases of Kaposi's sarcoma in Port au Prince provides circumstantial evidence for this theory. If KS, the cancer that has been found among AIDS patients in this country, is a marker for AIDS, then a recent outbreak of KS could signal that AIDS also existed in Haiti. Americans who had sexual contact with Haitians while on vacation there could have brought the disease to the United States.

A CDC study provided additional evidence that AIDS was a communicable disease. The investigators looked at the records of 170 gay men. Fifty had AIDS; the remaining 120 functioned as "con-

Cases of Karposi syndrome opportunistic infection by specific diagnosis, year of onset, sex, and sexual orientation, United States, 1978–1982

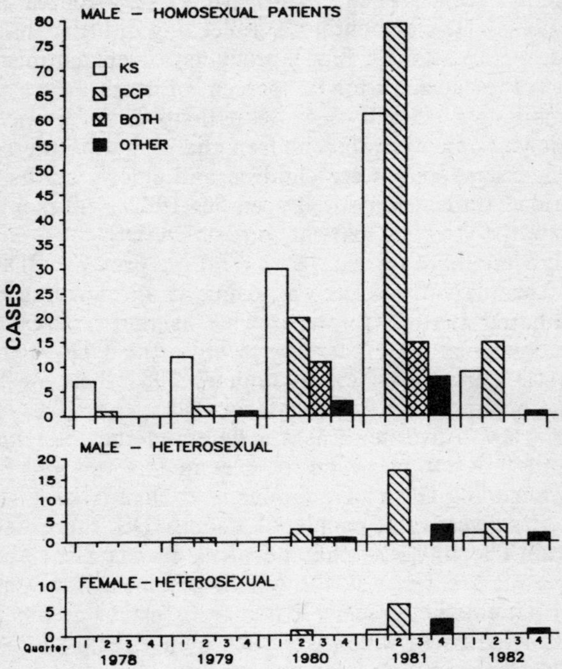

Reported cases of Pneumocystis carinii *pneumonia in previously healthy persons, June 1, 1981–May 28, 1982, United States*

		Race			Case-fatality	
	Total	White	Black	Hispanic	ratio	IV-Drug Use†
Homosexual men*	118	80	22	15	51%	11/80 (14%)
Heterosexual men*	26	8	11	6	35%	17/26 (65%)
Heterosexual women*	8	1	4	2	50%	4/7 (57%)

*Race data lacking for 1 case

†Data not available on all cases

Source: U.S. Department of Health and Human Services, Public Health Service, Centers for Disease Control, Morbidity and Mortality Weekly Report, Vol. 31, No. 22, June 11, 1982.

trols"—they were similar in age and background but didn't have AIDS. The study found that AIDS patients had a significantly higher number of different sexual partners and a history of many more sexually transmitted diseases than did the "controls." AIDS sufferers had an average of 61 different sexual contacts per year, twice the number of contacts of the gay men who remained healthy. Those who ran the greatest risk of acquiring known STDs also ran the greatest risk of acquiring AIDS.

It isn't a moral judgment to say that AIDS is linked to having many sexual contacts. It reflects a reality about all STDs. The more partners one has, the higher the chances become that someone will have a transmissible disease. And as the concentration of a disease within a community rises, the odds that any given sexual encounter will transmit an infection increase. While there is an element of chance that one might acquire an STD from any single contact, the likelihood increases with the number of partners and the proportion of infected individuals in the community.

A CDC report on June 18, 1982, gave additional weight to the communicable nature of AIDS. There was a cluster of 19 cases from Los Angeles and Orange Counties. Of the 19 patients, nine had had contact with at least one other patient and four had had contact with more than one AIDS patient.

Even though all the evidence suggests that AIDS is contagious, there is no evidence to suggest that casual contact, such as hugging, can spread the disease. There is also nothing to suggest that AIDS can be spread through the air, by sneezing or coughing. And, even though AIDS seems to be spread through sexual contact, most lovers of AIDS patients have not come down with the disease. No one really knows how contagious the disease is. But given the stakes involved, people should make every effort to protect themselves and others.

What exactly is AIDS? Because it is new, its cause uncertain, and its manifestations so varied, AIDS is difficult to define. The "working definition"—the definition used by doctors who are trying to unravel the problem—may need to be revised as the problem becomes better understood.

For the moment, the CDC counts only those with the following characteristics as having AIDS: Patients must be less than 60 years old, have biopsy-proven Kaposi's sarcoma or culture-proven opportunistic infections (infections that don't strike people with healthy immune systems), and they cannot have any other known reason for immune suppression. Only those patients who meet this strict definition are now being counted by the CDC. Persons who have the seemingly related syndrome of swollen nodes and immune abnormalities, but who don't have cancer or a rare infection, don't enter into the tally.

THE IMMUNE SYSTEM

While it is the infections and cancer that the CDC uses to recognize AIDS, the real problem lies in the workings of the immune system. In order to understand AIDS, one has to know what the immune system should do and how it malfunctions in this disease.

The immune system is the body's internal defense against infection and cancer, a sort of vigilante network that separates "self" from "nonself" and destroys what it perceives as "nonself." Infectious agents, cells that have been transformed by infection or cancer, and cells derived from other people during organ transplantation all fall into the "nonself" category. Occasionally, the immune system errs in its perception of "nonself" and attacks normal tissues, causing what are known as the "autoimmune" disorders— such as rheumatoid arthritis or lupus.

The white blood cells are the immune system's main weapon in the fight to protect the body's integrity. Of the two main types of white blood cells, the "neutrophils" and the "lymphocytes," the lymphocytes function as the system's intelligence; they coordinate the defense. Without belittling their importance, the neutrophils function more as a cleanup crew, chewing up bacteria and cellular debris.

Lymphocytes provide two lines of defense. The first destroys bacteria and viruses before they enter the cells. This is the job of the "humoral" immune system. The B lymphocytes (B stands for bone marrow–derived) perform this function by making antibodies against infectious agents. The second line of defense copes with infectious organisms once they have entered the cells. This is the job of T lymphocytes (T stands for thymus-derived) and is known as the cellular immune system. In addition to dealing with infection, the cellular immune system does "cancer surveillance"—looking for malignant cells and destroying them—and also is responsible for transplant rejection.

B and T lymphocytes have separate functions, but they are interrelated. For example, T cells stimulate B cells to make antibodies. In practical terms, B cells primarily protect the body against bacterial and viral invasion. T lymphocytes defend the body once the bacteria or viruses have entered the cell and are the main protection against parasites and fungi.

In AIDS, it is the cellular immune system, the one run by T lymphocytes, that fails. This is what makes patients susceptible to rare infections and to cancer. The humoral immune system, comprised of B cells, seems to work normally.

Many studies have been done to determine the exact nature of the immune defect in AIDS. The one consistent finding throughout these studies is that patients have an abnormally low ratio of helper to suppressor T cells. Helper and suppressor cells are two subsets of T cells; helper cells increase the immune response and suppressor cells decrease it. The normal ratio of helper to suppressor cells is between 1.75 and 2.1; the ratio in AIDS patients is less than 1 to 1. In the scientific literature, the helper/suppressor ratio is often called the Leu3/Leu2 or OKT4/OKT8 ratio; these are different terms for the same finding.

Other abnormalities of immune function have been found by many studies but are not as consistently present as the abnormal helper/suppressor ratio. There may be a decrease in the total number of white blood cells, the total number of lymphocytes, or only of the T lymphocytes. In some laboratory studies, T cells from AIDS patients do not proliferate in response to substances that normally make T cells divide, such as phytohemagglutinin, a kidney-bean extract. Some studies also report a decrease in "natural killer cell" (NK) activity. NK cells are thought to be related to T cells and to destroy tumor cells.

AIDS isn't the only disease that impairs cellular immunity. Some people are born with a defective immune system; they have a "congenital" immune deficiency syndrome. Other people develop the problem later in life; they have an "acquired" immune deficiency. Viral infections, cancer, and the drugs used to prevent transplant rejections and treat autoimmune disorders can all suppress the cellular immune system. But once the infection subsides, the drugs are stopped, or the cancer cured, the patient regains normal immunity. This is the opposite of what happens in AIDS; patients don't recover normal cellular immunity. This is what makes AIDS so deadly.

Without spontaneous recovery of immune function, the vulnerability to infection and cancer persists.

Some doctors think that for every gay man with full-blown AIDS, there are 5 to 20 more who have milder but related immune abnormalities. Depending on what happens to these men, the number of AIDS patients could go much higher than current figures suggest. Several studies are under way to determine what is likely to happen to those men who now fall into this gray area. Preliminary results show recovery of normal immunity in some and progression to AIDS in others. It is still too early to draw definite conclusions. What seems to be true is that many gay men who feel healthy have immune abnormalities similar to the ones found in AIDS. But it simply isn't known whether they have a forerunner of AIDS or a much milder case of the disease.

WHAT CAUSES AIDS?

The theories about what causes AIDS have shifted in popularity since the problem was first discovered. The major current theory is that an infectious agent, probably a virus, causes AIDS. Other theories may explain why certain people are more vulnerable than others to the infection. But until a cause of AIDS can be isolated in the laboratory, explanations are really theories. These are the theories.

The Viral Theory

The analogy of AIDS to hepatitis B, with apparently similar distributions and modes of transmission, is good circumstantial evidence that AIDS is also caused by a virus.

Two members of the herpesvirus family have come under suspicion. Cytomegalovirus (CMV) and Epstein-Barr virus (EBV) can suppress the immune system, even causing the abnormal helper/suppressor T cell ratio that is seen in AIDS. Both viruses have also been linked to cancer; EBV is linked to Burkitt's lymphoma, common in Africa, and CMV has been found in the lesions of Kaposi's sarcoma. Gay men are often exposed to both viruses, as shown by the frequent presence in their blood of antibodies to these viruses. One study found that 90 percent of gay men had CMV antibody, compared to 54 percent of straight men. CMV can also be transmitted for a long time after someone becomes infected. The virus has been found to persist in the urine and semen for as long as one year.

Of the two viruses, it is primarily CMV that is thought to possibly cause AIDS, because the virus is so common and because it is associated with KS and with some of the rare infections that AIDS patients get. But there are several problems with the CMV theory. One, the virus has been around for a long time without causing AIDS. This might mean that there is a new strain of the virus, which is now causing AIDS, but experiments have failed to show that a single strain of CMV is common to all AIDS patients. It would be unlikely for many new strains to suddenly appear. A second problem with the theory is that not all of the heterosexual AIDS patients have had CMV antibodies. Since it is probable that AIDS is caused by the same agent in everyone, the lack of evidence of CMV infection in some patients suggests that CMV is not the cause.

Another virus that has been invoked as a possible cause of AIDS is the human T-cell leukemia virus (HTLV). This virus causes an aggressive leukemia in adults. It can be transmitted through blood and it is endemic in the Caribbean. With the recent cluster of Haitian cases, this provides a geographic link between the virus and AIDS.

Whatever virus causes AIDS, it seems to have an incubation period that varies from six months to two years. This information was derived from cases where the date of exposure could be estimated and where the onset of illness was known.

Since the epidemic of immune suppression is new, scientists are wondering whether they may be dealing with a new virus. It is of interest that a case similar to AIDS in many ways was reported in a British medical journal more than 20 years ago. In the *Lancet* of October 29, 1960, doctors described a young man with oral and anal ulcers who died rapidly of overwhelming *Pneumocystis* and CMV infection. On the surface at least, this sounds much like AIDS.

The Antigen-Overload Theory

Antigens are substances that the body recognizes as foreign and that stimulate the immune system to make antibodies. Unlike the infection theory, which implicates one organism as the cause of AIDS, the antigen-overload theory is that multiple infections have a cumulative effect of overwhelming the immune system. The body doesn't get the adequate respite of infection-free periods needed to maintain a healthy immune system. While it is true that most gay men with AIDS have a history of many STDs, and that intravenous drug users and hemophiliacs are exposed to many viruses, there are gaps in the antigen-overload explanation. Not all individuals have a history of multiple infections, nor do they have laboratory evidence of having had similar infections.

The Drug Theory

This theory implicates "recreational" drugs as a cause of immune suppression. Intravenous heroin is known to alter cellular immunity. Marijuana, amphetamines, and cocaine have been suspected of interfering with the immune system. But the drugs that have come under greatest attack in this epidemic are the "poppers," amyl, butyl, and iso-butyl nitrite.

Taken to enhance orgasm, relax the anal sphincter, and induce a sense of well-being, butyl and iso-butyl nitrites are sold as room odorizers or liquid incense. Amyl nitrite, which serves the same purposes, has required a prescription since 1968, but it, too, is widely available. These drugs already have a long list of adverse side effects. They can cause serious blood disorders, such as a Heinz-body hemolytic anemia—the body destroys its own red blood cells—and methemoglobinemia—a form of hemoglobin that no longer delivers oxygen. Poppers are skin irritants; they also dilate blood vessels and cause a rapid heart rate—both of which stress the heart's pumping abilities. The nitrites can be fatal if swallowed, and amyl nitrite is a known mutagen, raising the question of whether it is carcinogenic. Now, poppers are suspected of also causing immune disturbances. Sixty percent of the gay men who have developed AIDS have used poppers repeatedly.

But the popper explanation of AIDS also has loopholes. Not all patients, either gay or straight, have used them. Poppers may simply be markers for a life-style that involves many sexual partners, a life-style that could account for increased exposure to an infectious agent. But even if poppers don't directly cause AIDS, they could make one more vulnerable to infection by lowering the immune defenses.

The Sperm Theory

This theory holds that sperm entering the bloodstream, through tears in the mucous lining of the rectum that are caused by anal intercourse, suppress the immune system. The body seems capable of making antibodies against sperm that cross-react with T lymphocytes and may inactivate T cells. Two findings support a link between sperm antibodies and immune suppression. The first is an experiment done by the National Cancer Institute which showed that mice who were injected with sperm into their veins had no cellular immunity 52 days after injection. The second line of evidence comes from the finding that many gay men with AIDS have had low sperm counts and high levels of sperm antibody; the sperm antibody would explain the low sperm counts and could contribute to the immune suppression that underlies AIDS.

While this theory may partially explain the immune disorders in gay men, it doesn't apply to many other AIDS patients. Since everyone probably develops AIDS for the same reason, it is unlikely that the sperm theory by itself could explain AIDS.

The Genetic Theory

This theory holds that individual differences in the immune system, which are genetically determined, render some people more susceptible than others to AIDS. Everyone has certain immune markers on the surface of his white blood cells. Known as HLA (human leukocyte antigens) markers, they are genetically determined and are used to decide whether an organ donor and transplant recipient are immunologically compatible. It is known that certain diseases are much more common in individuals with certain HLA types. Now it has been found that 60 percent of AIDS patients with Kaposi's sarcoma have the HLA marker DR5. The incidence of this marker in the general population is only 12 to 23 percent. Thus patients with HLA type DR5 would be more likely to get KS; whether they are more likely to get AIDS in general isn't yet known.

SYMPTOMS

The symptoms of AIDS fall into two categories: They may be due to a specific disease that is an expression of AIDS, such as the cough of *Pneumocystis carinii* pneumonia; or they may reflect the underlying illness, such as the lymph-node swelling seen in many AIDS patients. The symptoms that follow are ones that should prompt medical attention but no single symptom is specific for AIDS. Given the stakes of the disease and the possibility that early treatment will improve the outcome, it is better to consult a doctor for what may turn out to be a minor problem than to worry about it in private, waiting for the problem to go away.

Fever

A fever of more than 100° F. that persists for weeks or months without an explanation is one sign of AIDS. The fever may occur daily or may be intermittent.

Weight Loss

An unexplained weight loss of more than 10 pounds or more than 10 percent of one's normal body weight within a two-month period should be looked into. Some AIDS patients have developed a "wasting syndrome," where they lose weight for no clear-cut reason.

Lymph-Node Swelling

Lymph nodes are found behind the ears, in the neck, under the chin, above the collarbone, under the armpits, next to the elbow, and in the groin. Lymph nodes also exist deep inside the body, but can't be detected on a physical examination. Many people have slightly swollen nodes in the groin without having anything wrong. However, swollen nodes in other areas imply disease—although not necessarily a serious disease. Significant lymph-node swelling, the sort that has been seen in AIDS, is defined as swelling that has lasted for more than three months and affects nodes in at least two areas of the body, excluding the groin. This sort of swelling can be caused by many things, including common infections and reactions to drugs; it does not automatically mean that someone has AIDS. But anyone who finds lumps on his body, which is what the swollen nodes feel like, should see his doctor.

Fatigue

Everyone goes through periods of feeling tired, and initially it may be hard to tell whether the degree of tiredness is truly abnormal. But AIDS patients often develop persistent, severe fatigue.

Diarrhea

Patients with severe diarrhea, or diarrhea that lasts for more than a week, should see their doctor to exclude a treatable cause. AIDS patients, however, can develop diarrhea that has no apparent cause.

Shortness of Breath and Dry Cough

These may be the earliest signs of *Pneumocystis* pneumonia. Unlike the usual bacterial pneumonias, which cause patients to cough up thick yellow or green sputum, PCP may cause much more subtle symptoms, such as shortness of breath during physical exertion and a cough that doesn't produce any sputum.

Oral Thrush

Patients may notice patches of white material inside their mouths which can be easily scraped off the surface. This may be thrush, a yeast infection caused by *Candida albicans*. If the infection spreads down the throat and into the esophagus, the tube that connects the throat to the stomach, patients may have pain when they swallow.

Skin Spots

The lesions of Kaposi's sarcoma are very varied. The typical ones are painless, purplish-brown spots that occur anywhere on the body. Patients with AIDS may also get painful, recurrent herpes ulcers near the mouth or anus.

Night Sweats

Patients with night sweats wake up drenched in the middle of the night. The bed may be so wet that they need to change the sheets. Night sweats are a classic symptom of tuberculosis, but they may also be a symptom of AIDS.

Neurological Problems

A wide variety of nervous-system problems have recently been found in AIDS patients. These vary from subtle psychiatric symptoms, such as personality changes and depression, to more severe ones, such as hallucinations. Patients may also develop memory loss and seizures.

DIAGNOSIS

The first step in diagnosing AIDS is thinking of it. The doctor must consider the possibility that AIDS might be causing the patient's symptoms. The diagnostic tests to be ordered then depend on the particular symptoms that the patient has and how sick he is. The evaluation of someone who has only a low-grade fever can begin in the doctor's office, but a patient who is very short of breath may well need to be hospitalized. The tests that are ordered are designed to ascertain whether the patient has any of the specific diseases associated with AIDS, such as KS or PCP, and to see whether he has the immune disorder associated with AIDS.

These are a few general guidelines about where to begin. More-specific tests will be described with the discussion of specific diseases.

Patients should try to document such symptoms as fevers and weight loss. This means actually writing down one's temperature and weight. This is very helpful for the doctor, who will have a better idea of how serious the situation really is.

All patients who are suspected of having AIDS should have a simple blood test known as a "complete blood count" or CBC. This reveals whether they are anemic; whether they have a normal level of white blood cells, including lymphocytes; and whether they have a normal number of platelets, the cells responsible for blood clotting. The CBC should also include a "differential" count of the white blood cells, which specifies how many of the total white blood cells are lymphocytes and neutrophils. Many AIDS patients have a low lymphocyte count in the face of otherwise normal CBCs.

The other simple test that can be done in the doctor's office is a "skin test." To see whether the cellular immune system is working well, a small amount of an "antigen" is injected into the skin of the forearm. A positive reaction, which means that someone has been exposed to the antigen before and that his immune system can react against it, shows up as redness and swelling at the injection site 24 to 72 hours after the injection. The tuberculosis skin test is a well-known example of this kind of test.

Virtually everyone with a normal cellular immune system reacts to at least one of the many antigens that are commonly used. A patient who doesn't react to any of them has something wrong with his immune system, although he may not have AIDS. A positive reaction also does not definitively exclude AIDS since a few patients have reacted to the skin tests. But "anergy"—the absence of a reaction to skin tests—is a very common finding in AIDS patients. Usually people have no response to four or five antigens before they are called "anergic."

If the results of these simple tests, the CBC and skin tests, are abnormal, more-sophisticated tests of immune function are usually called for. A blood sample is analyzed for the ratio of helper-to-suppressor T cells, and the T cells will be examined to see whether they proliferate normally in response to certain chemical stimuli. Although these tests are simple from the patient's standpoint, they are very time-consuming in the laboratory and therefore expensive. In addition, they are new tests and must be done with great accuracy in a good laboratory for the results to be meaningful.

These tests are appropriate for diagnosing patients suspected of having AIDS and for studies that are trying to unravel the mystery of AIDS. Preliminary results of these studies have shown that many apparently healthy gay men have abnormal helper/suppressor cell ratios; one study has suggested that some men regained normal ratios after curtailing the number of different sexual partners. Eventually, such studies will help elucidate how AIDS and the immune system behave.

But these sophisticated tests of the immune system are not, at the moment, meant to be screening tests—contrary to what some commercial laboratories are now suggesting. Screening tests are usually meant to find disease at an early stage in patients who don't have symptoms, and, by detecting disease, hopefully alter its outcome through early treatment. Good screening tests should also be specific—positive results should mean that a patient has the disease. These tests of the immune system do not meet either criterion: there is no treatment for the immune abnormality and the immune abnormality, by itself, does not mean that someone has AIDS. A new simpler test that measures the level of the hormone thymosin alpha-1 and that may be more specific for AIDS is under investigation as a possible screening test.

Patients with swollen lymph nodes should be tested for the common, non-AIDS causes of this problem, which are discussed in the next section, "Diseases Associated with AIDS." Even if no cause is found, the doctor may decide to check the nodes once a month for three months, recording their number and size. If they haven't gone away by then, a biopsy may be in order. This can be done on an outpatient basis, under local anesthesia. But the three-month waiting period is not a hard-and-fast rule, and a doctor may have good reasons for deciding to do a biopsy earlier.

Any patient who has shortness of breath and a dry cough, who might have AIDS, should have a prompt chest X-ray. These symptoms could mean PCP, and this infection should be treated with antibiotics as soon as possible. Patients with diarrhea should be tested for infections that cause diarrhea in non-AIDS patients. These tests are fully discussed in the chapter "GI Blues." Patients with skin spots that could possibly be KS should have a biopsy.

DISEASES ASSOCIATED WITH AIDS

Technically, AIDS is a syndrome rather than a disease. Like many medical syndromes, AIDS has a group of symptoms that distinguish it from other illnesses but lacks an identifiable cause.

The diseases associated with AIDS, which stem from the underlying immune abnormality, are myriad but can be divided into four basic categories. The two main ones are infections and cancers. The third is a poorly understood phenomenon of generalized lymph-node swelling that may turn out to be an early stage of AIDS or a milder version of it. The fourth disease belongs to a group of problems called "autoimmune" disorders, disorders caused by an overactive immune system.

Although each of the diseases that have been associated with AIDS will be described separately, this doesn't mean that patients get only one at a time. Many people have had KS *and* a rare infection, and many people have several infections simultaneously.

The diseases discussed below are those that have been found in AIDS patients, but the list does not include every disease known to occur in immune-suppressed patients. Such a list would be too long, and would include diseases that have not been seen in AIDS patients. It is conceivable, however, that the list of diseases seen with AIDS will expand or change with time.

Two of the diseases, the infection *Pneumocystis carinii* pneumonia and the cancer Kaposi's sarcoma, are by far the most common problems; 51 percent of AIDS patients have had PCP, 28 percent have had KS, and 7 percent have had both PCP and KS. Fourteen percent of patients have had other "opportunistic infections"—rare infections that usually don't afflict people with normal immune systems. Patients with other problems, which are assumed to be part of the spectrum of AIDS, are omitted from these statistics because they do not fit the narrow CDC definition of AIDS. But the fact remains that PCP and KS are by far the most common illnesses.

The mortality rate of AIDS is frightening, but it is variable depending, in part, on what disease someone has. The overall mortality rate is said to be 36 percent. Patients with only KS fare best, with a mortality rate of 20 percent; those with PCP and KS have the worst prognosis, with a mortality rate of 48 percent. In between are those with PCP alone, who have a 41-percent mortality rate, and those with other infections, whose mortality rate is 44 percent.

Although these are the mortality rates quoted by the CDC in March 1983, AIDS is such a new problem that it is hard to tell what these statistics really mean. For mortality rates to be useful, they have to be linked to time, and these rates are not. To say that a disease has a mortality rate of 5 percent after one year but a 50-percent mortality rate after 5 years implies a very different outcome from saying that a disease has a 5-percent mortality rate after one year and a 6-percent mortality rate after five years. In the first instance, the patient who survives for one year cannot be reassured that he is likely to survive the next four; in the second case, a patient can, on a statistical basis, reasonably expect to survive the next four years once he has lived through the first year. When the survival rates for AIDS are linked to time, the implications are grim—75 percent of patients diagnosed before 1982 have died. One hopes that greater awareness of the disease, by physicians and the public, will lead to earlier diagnosis and better results from treatment. The ultimate hope is that the cause of and cure for AIDS will soon be discovered.

Infections

Opportunistic infections are, by definition, ones that afflict patients with poorly functioning immune systems. While healthy people are often exposed to these organisms, their immune systems usually avert serious infection. The diseases that follow are found in patients with cellular immune problems. Because AIDS patients have normal humoral immune systems, they don't have particular difficulty with the common bacterial infections such as pneumococcal pneumonia.

PROTOZOAN INFECTIONS

Pneumocystis carinii Pneumonia (PCP)

There is still some doubt about the classification of *Pneumocystis carinii,* but it is probably a protozoan, a one-celled parasite, that causes pneumonia. Studies show that two-thirds of children have antibodies against *P. carinii* by the age of four, suggesting that most people are likely to be exposed to *Pneumocystis.* The organism is virtually ubiquitous; it has been found in people and animals across five continents.

Pneumocystis enters the body through the lungs, but it isn't clear how patients with lowered immune defenses become sick from it. It isn't known whether they have caught a new infection or whether the infection has been lying dormant in the body and now runs rampant because their defenses are down. The other question about PCP is its relation to cytomegalovirus, since patients are often infected with the protozoan and this virus simultaneously. The frequency with which these two infections occur together in immune-suppressed patients seems to suggest more than coincidence.

Pneumocystis carinii pneumonia is a relatively new disease in the United States; the first case was reported in 1955. Until the recent outbreak of PCP in AIDS patients, this infection had not been seen in people thought to have normal immune systems. The appearance of PCP was, in fact, the tip-off that a profound alteration of the body's immune function was the basis of the problem now known as AIDS.

Before patients develop the specific symptoms of PCP, they often have nonspecific complaints: fever, fatigue, and weight loss. These are followed by the classic symptoms of PCP: shortness of breath and a cough that is either dry or produces small amounts of white sputum. Some patients also have sharp chest pain when they inhale deeply.

The diagnosis of PCP begins with a chest X-ray, which characteristically shows a patchy pneumonia in both lungs. An arterial blood sample is often drawn for a "blood gas," a test that reflects how well the lungs are able to deliver oxygen to the bloodstream.

If PCP looks likely, the next step is to find the protozoan. This can be done either by bronchoscopy, in which a tube is passed through the mouth into the lungs, or by an "open lung biopsy," an operation in which a piece of lung tissue is removed. The advantages of bronchoscopy are that it avoids the pain and general anesthesia of surgery. The disadvantages are that it may miss the area of infection and that it is harder to control bleeding complications if they arise. Once the lung sample is obtained, it is stained with a special methenamine-silver stain and examined under the microscope.

Two drugs are used to treat PCP. The first is a widely used combination antibiotic, trimethoprim/sulfamethoxazole, which goes under the trade name of Bactrim or Septra. In the high doses used to treat PCP (20mg/100mg per kilogram, divided into 4 oral or intravenous doses and given daily for 14 days), the side effects include blood disorders, rashes, and mental confusion. But this drug causes much milder problems than the alternative, pentamidine. This is the drug that was first available for PCP and the one that is now used if Bactrim fails. It is only available through the CDC. A daily injection of 4mg per kilogram for 14 days is the usual dose. Pentamidine can cause serious liver and kidney impairment and reactions at the injection site. Patients may be treated with one drug at a time or with both simultaneously.

AIDS patients who have had PCP or are felt to be at risk for PCP may be given a low, oral dose of Bactrim or Septra to prevent future infections.

Without treatment, the mortality of PCP is greater than 90 percent. With treatment, this figure drops to 25–50 percent. But while AIDS patients may recover from a bout of PCP, they remain vulnerable to future problems.

Toxoplasmosis

Toxoplasma gondii is also a protozoan that commonly affects Americans and has a worldwide distribution. Unlike *Pneumocystis, Toxoplasma* does cause symptoms in healthy persons, but it doesn't cause the severe nervous-system disorders that are seen in immune-suppressed patients.

Toxoplasma is usually acquired through an oral route—by eating undercooked meat or substances that have been contaminated with cat feces. Cats are a major reservoir of this infection. But *Toxoplasma* can also be acquired through other routes, through blood transfusions and transplanted organs. Like *Pneumocystis, Toxoplasma* infection in immune-suppressed patients is so frequently associated with simultaneous CMV infection that it seems more than a matter of coincidence. But it isn't known how the two are related.

Healthy adults who get toxoplasmosis get a mild, mononucleosis-like illness, with fever, swollen glands, and malaise. But immune-suppressed patients, such as those with AIDS, get a life-threatening brain infection. The symptoms are headaches, severe lethargy, seizures, vomiting, and fever. *Toxoplasma* can also infect the heart and lungs, but the infection is usually discovered because of brain-related symptoms.

Toxoplasmosis can be diagnosed both by blood tests and by tests looking for the protozoan. Positive blood tests show either a very high antibody level or an antibody level that increases during the course of the illness. The common places to look for the protozoan are the brain, the lymph nodes, and the fluid that surrounds the brain and spinal column. It is easiest to biopsy a lymph node or examine the fluid obtained by doing a spinal tap. Under local anesthesia, a needle is inserted into the low back to withdraw a sample of the fluid that bathes the spinal cord. Patients with certain neurological signs will probably have a special X-ray of the brain, known as a CAT scan. If this shows an abscess, a pocket of infection, a brain biopsy will be done to confirm that *Toxoplasma* is the cause.

The 80-percent mortality rate of untreated *Toxoplasma* brain infections is reduced by using a combination of two drugs, pyrimethamine and sulfadiazine, for at least one month. The main side effects of treatment are a low white-blood-cell count and low platelet count. Although 80 percent of patients are said to respond to treatment, the mortality rate remains high.

Cryptosporidiosis

Cryptosporidium is a protozoan that is more familiar to veterinarians for causing disease among animals, particularly calves, than it is to doctors for causing illness among humans. But on November 12,

1982, the CDC reported that 21 AIDS patients had developed cryptosporidiosis.

Diarrhea is the only symptom. Persons with normal immune systems can develop the infection, but the diarrhea goes away after one or two weeks. AIDS patients, however, can develop chronic diarrhea, with as many as 25 watery bowel movements a day. Usually the diagnosis is made by biopsying the small or large intestine, which can be done through a long tube that is passed through the mouth or anus. A special stool test has recently become available, however, that may eliminate the need for a biopsy in the diagnosis of cryptosporidiosis.

Many drugs have been tested against the infection, but the CDC reports that none is clearly effective. Treatment consists primarily of replacing the lost fluid and supplying adequate nutrition.

Although the death rate in this group of 21 patients was nearly 70 percent, *Cryptosporidium* was not thought to be the direct cause of death in any case. But it may have been a contributing factor by causing malnutrition.

VIRAL INFECTIONS

Cytomegalovirus

Cytomegalovirus (CMV) can cause a transient mononucleosis-like illness, with fever, swollen lymph nodes, and malaise in healthy persons. But in immune-suppressed patients, such as those with AIDS, CMV causes a widespread, devastating illness. Although the lung is the most common site of infection, CMV can spread to almost any organ.

The virus belongs to the herpesvirus family. It is transmitted in the semen, urine, blood, and saliva. People commonly get CMV infections through sexual contact and blood transfusions. Because the virus can persist in the urine and semen for a year after exposure, there is a great potential for spread of CMV.

As mentioned earlier, some investigators think that CMV may be a cause of AIDS. The virus is spread the same way that AIDS appears to be spread; it causes abnormal helper/suppressor T-cell ratios; and it is very common among gay men. Surveys in New York and California show that over 90 percent of gay men tested had past or current CMV infections.

But CMV infection may be the result rather than the cause of AIDS. Other patients who are immune-suppressed, such as kidney-transplant patients, are very prone to CMV infection. No one knows whether the lowered defenses make someone vulnerable to a new infection or whether they permit a virus that has been lying dormant in the body to now go uncontrolled.

AIDS patients most often develop a lung infection, but hepatitis and gastrointestinal ulcers are also relatively common. Specific symptoms depend on where the infection has spread. Most patients also have generalized symptoms such as fever and malaise.

The diagnosis is made both by blood tests, showing a high antibody level or one that rises during the course of the illness, and by cultures of the throat, lung tissue, semen, or urine.

There is no effective treatment for CMV. The available antiviral drugs don't seem to work against this virus.

Herpes

Two members of the herpes family—herpes simplex and herpes zoster—can cause severe symptoms in patients whose immune systems are impaired. Both cause milder versions of the same symptoms in otherwise healthy people.

Herpes simplex, the virus that causes cold sores and anogenital blisters, has caused persistent, severe oral and perianal ulcers in gay men with AIDS. The ulcers are painful, and the anal ones are associated with the symptoms of colitis: rectal bleeding, abdominal pain, fever, and weight loss.

The appearance of the lesions will suggest the diagnosis, but this should be confirmed by culturing the ulcers. A cotton swab is rubbed along the ulcer and sent to the laboratory.

Acyclovir, a newly available drug whose trade name is Zovirax, is the treatment of choice. This is the same medication that is used to treat ordinary genital herpes, but in immune-suppressed patients the intravenous form, rather than the ointment, is used.

Herpes zoster causes a skin eruption colloquially known as "shingles." It can occur in anyone, but patients with poorly functioning immune systems get longer-lasting and more widespread lesions.

The appearance of the spots varies quite a bit, from red spots to oozing blisters to black scabs. The spots may or may not be painful, and pain in the area may precede the appearance of the rash. The classic distribution of shingles is due to the fact that the virus infects a sensory nerve, causing a skin eruption along the nerve's pathway. Because the right and left side of the body have separate nerves, the rash usually affects only one side.

Herpes zoster is diagnosed by the appearance of the skin lesions and their distinctive distribution. While there is no specific treatment for herpes zoster in patients with normal immune systems, the antiviral drug vidarabine may benefit those who are immune-suppressed.

FUNGAL INFECTIONS

Candidiasis

Candida albicans is a normal inhabitant of mucous membranes and skin. Except for an occasional rash in the warm, moist body folds of the groin and armpits, healthy men don't develop symptoms from *Candida*. AIDS patients, however, are often troubled by symptoms.

Thrush, a *Candida* infection of the mouth, is very common and may be an early warning sign of AIDS. Patients get a white substance in their mouths that has a consistency akin to cottage cheese and that can be easily scraped off the surface. Sometimes thrush causes a sore throat. But more serious problems arise if the infection spreads down the esophagus, the tube that connects the throat to the stomach. Patients develop chest pain and difficulty in swallowing. And the infection can spread into the bloodstream.

The oral infection is easy to diagnose and treat. The cheesy substance can be cultured and looked at under the microscope, and the infection is treated with a liquid medication, nystatin, that rarely has any side effects.

Infection of the esophagus is harder to diagnose and to treat. The diagnosis requires either endoscopy, in which a tube is passed through the mouth into the esophagus, or an X-ray taken after the patient has swallowed barium, a chalky liquid. With endoscopy, the doctor is able to see the white, cheesy substance and to take a sample for culture. The X-ray shows a ragged lining of the esophagus that is characteristic of candidal esophagitis.

Ketoconazole, a new oral drug, is used to treat the esophagitis. Although it commonly causes nausea, its side effects are minor compared to those of other antifungal drugs. These drugs, amphotericin B and flucytosine, may still be needed if the infection does not respond to ketoconazole or spreads beyond the esophagus.

Cryptococcosis

Although *Cryptococcus neoformans* enters the body through the lungs, the main problem that it causes for AIDS patients is meningitis, an inflammation of the tissues surrounding the brain and spinal column.

Patients get a severe headache, stiff neck, fever, and become stuporous. They may also develop double vision and facial weakness.

The diagnosis is made by doing a spinal tap. The fluid is then stained with India ink and looked at under the microscope. It is also cultured for *Cryptococcus* and biochemically tested for this fungus.

The treatment of cryptococcosis is difficult because there is a high relapse rate and because the antibiotics have serious side effects. Amphotericin B and flucytosine are usually used in combination. The flucytosine helps reduce the amount of amphotericin that is needed, an important consideration since amphotericin causes fever and kidney damage. Treatment usually requires 6 to 12 weeks of intravenous medication.

Histoplasmosis

Histoplasma capsulatum is very common in the mideastern region of the United States. Healthy adults may get a flu-like illness or pneumonia from *Histoplasma,* but AIDS patients get a widespread infection that can involve the liver, lymph nodes, bone marrow, skin, gastrointestinal tract, and brain.

Tissue biopsy is the way to diagnose histoplasmosis. Samples are usually taken from the bone marrow or liver during procedures that are done under local anesthesia with the patient lying in bed. The samples are then examined under the microscope and cultured. The infection is treated with amphotericin B.

BACTERIAL INFECTIONS

Mycobacterial Infections

The best-known member of this family is *Mycobacterium tuberculosis,* the bug that causes TB. Patients whose cellular immune systems malfunction are very susceptible to reactivation of TB that has been lying dormant in the body.

But a much rarer mycobacterium, *Mycobacterium avium-intracellulare,* has emerged with unusual frequency among AIDS patients. Although both types of mycobacteria cause pneumonia, lymph-node swelling, weight loss, and fever, and both are treated with the same antibiotics, there are important differences. TB can occur in healthy persons; *M. avium-intracellulare* occurs only in patients with underlying illnesses. While TB pneumonia is easy to cure with two antibiotics, *M. avium-intracellulare* pneumonia often persists despite treatment with four or five antibiotics simultaneously.

The diagnosis of both diseases begins with a sputum sample, usually obtained by having the patient cough. The sample is then treated with a special stain, known as the "acid-fast stain." This test takes only minutes to do, but it can't distinguish between *M. tuberculosis* and *M. avium-intracellulare.* A culture can make this distinction, but it may take as long as one month to obtain an answer.

In addition to two of the drugs that are ordinarily used to treat TB—isoniazid (called INH for short) and rifampin or ethambutol—*M. avium-intracellulare* also requires streptomycin and ethionamide. Treatment continues for at least 18 months and the results are variable. A new drug, Ansamycin, is currently being investigated.

Legionnaires' Disease

The bacterium, *Legionella pneumophila,* that causes Legionnaires' disease was discovered after the Philadelphia outbreak of 1976. Although it can cause pneumonia in anyone, the evidence suggests that immune-suppressed patients are particularly vulnerable to infection.

Two types of symptoms are rarely seen with other bacterial pneumonias yet are commonly associated with Legionnaires' disease. The first is abdominal: pain and watery diarrhea that occur at the beginning of the illness. The second is neurological: patients become confused and disoriented.

This unusual constellation of pneumonia with intestinal and nervous-system disorders is the basis for suspecting Legionnaires' disease. The diagnosis is usually confirmed by blood tests that show either a very high antibody level or a rising level. Unlike most bacteria, *Legionella* is very difficult to culture.

The infection is treated with two weeks of erythromycin.

CANCERS

Kaposi's Sarcoma (KS)

One month after the CDC reported that there had been an outbreak of an unusual infection among gay men, the CDC announced that a rare cancer, Kaposi's sarcoma (KS), was also being seen. Since the summer of 1981, KS has been transformed from an obscure disease to a problem of epidemic proportions.

After *Pneumocystis* pneumonia, KS is the most widespread disease associated with AIDS. By March 1983, nearly 30 percent of the 1240 patients with AIDS had KS. The incidence of this cancer was more than 100 times the number of cases that were expected in young patients. The National Cancer Institute established a special task force to study KS, which had become a new problem even though it wasn't a new disease.

Kaposi's sarcoma was discovered in 1872 by a Hungarian physician, Moritz Kaposi. The first international meeting on KS was held 90 years later in Uganda, where KS is common. In contrast to the United States and Western Europe where KS is rare, it causes nearly 10 percent of all cancers in certain parts of Africa.

Although KS can be described and diagnosed with certainty, the exact nature of the tumor isn't known. It probably comes from a cell that lines blood-vessel walls, but some investigators think it may be caused by a more primitive cell that can turn itself into a variety of cells as it matures. No one has actually been able to prove what the cell of origin is in KS. Unlike cancers that start from a single malignant cell and then metastasize or spread to other parts of the body, the cancerous transformation of KS occurs in many cells, arising *de novo* in different parts of the body.

While the variety of groups affected by AIDS has increased, KS has remained primarily a problem for gay men with AIDS. A few cases have been reported in male, heterosexual drug users, and by March 1983 a couple of women also seemed to have developed KS. But by and large, the heterosexual AIDS patients are getting rare infections and not KS.

The reason for this skewed distribution isn't known, but the link between KS and both CMV infection and genetic makeup could play a part. KS has been linked to CMV by finding parts of the virus within the tumor cells. If there turns out to be a cause-and-effect relationship between CMV and KS, then the high rates of CMV infection among gay men might explain why it is mainly gay men with AIDS who are getting KS. The link between genes and KS is supported by the finding that a certain genetic marker, the HLA-DR5 antigen, occurs in 60 percent of the gay men who have developed KS. Only 12 to 23 percent of the general population have the DR5 antigen. It is also noteworthy that KS, as the disease was known before the outbreak of AIDS, was already ten times more common among men than women.

Before KS became part of AIDS, the cancer was known to afflict three particular groups: young African men, elderly Western men, and patients whose immune systems were suppressed by either disease or medical treatment. Although the tumor looks the same under the microscope in each instance, the disease actually behaves differently in each group.

African men, especially those who live in the equatorial regions of Kenya and Uganda, tend to get the cancer at an early age—usually before they are 20. KS accounts for 9 percent of all cancers in this part of the world. The disease affects many internal organs, including the lymph nodes, gastrointestinal tract, lungs, and heart, and is usually fatal within three years. Although women do get KS in Africa, it is nine times more common in men.

KS was a much rarer problem in the West. Until the AIDS epidemic, the annual incidence was only .02 to .06 cases per 100,000 persons in the United States, meaning that there were between 40 and 120 cases diagnosed each year. These cases occurred in elderly men and immune-suppressed patients.

Elderly men are usually in their sixties at the time of diagnosis and usually of Mediterranean or Jewish background. Unlike the African version, which affects internal organs and tends to be fatal, these elderly men get skin tumors—painless, purplish-brown spots that are concentrated on the legs and feet. Their KS is rarely fatal. They survive an average of eight to thirteen years after diagnosis, usually dying of other diseases related to old age. But they do have a higher-than-expected rate of developing a second type of cancer, perhaps suggesting that they, like AIDS patients, have some immunologic impairment predisposing them to cancer. While women do get this version of KS, men are ten to fifteen times more likely to do so.

The other group of KS patients in the United States are those with impaired immune systems. Kidney-transplant patients, who take medication to prevent organ rejection—medication that works by dampening the immune system so that it doesn't reject the "nonself" kidney—have a high rate of KS. Immunosuppressive drugs are started at the time of transplantation and the cancer develops an average of 16 months later.

When transplant patients get KS, the illness resembles the African variety, spreading rapidly and affecting the internal organs. But when the drugs that suppress the immune system are stopped, the disease often goes into spontaneous remission. KS is clearly a cancer that appears when defenses are down and may disappear if defenses can be restored.

The disease that has emerged in AIDS patients, who are now the fourth group at risk for KS, has features of all three previous versions. Overwhelmingly, patients are young men, and both the skin and the internal organs are affected. The disease has a high mortality rate—20 percent, according to the CDC—and appears in conjunction with an immune problem. Unlike the situation in transplant patients, however, there is no way to remedy the immune problem.

The symptoms of KS include spots on the skin that usually don't hurt or itch. The spots vary from light pink to reddish-brown to purple. They can be very large or so small that they are dismissed as bug bites, and may be flat or raised. Unlike the elderly patients with KS, whose spots are restricted to the legs and feet, AIDS patients can develop them anywhere. KS lesions have been found in the mouth, in the eyes, behind the ears, on the torso and the limbs, and near the anus.

AIDS patients with KS frequently have generalized symptoms such as fever, weight loss, and lymph-node swelling that may even precede the appearance of skin lesions. Patients who have these general symptoms are more likely to have widespread KS.

When KS affects the internal organs, it most often involves one or more of the following organs: lymph nodes, lungs, stomach, liver, spleen, and intestine.

The diagnosis is made by doing a tissue biopsy. Skin lesions are the easiest because of their surface location. Enlarged lymph nodes from the neck or armpits can also be biopsied in a doctor's office, but they may show nonspecific changes. Two additional tests may be done to see whether any of the lymph nodes that lie deep within the body are enlarged. The first is a lymphangiogram, in which a dye is injected into the lymph system and then X-rays taken; the second is a CAT scan of the abdomen, which is a new type of X-ray.

KS lesions in the intestine cannot be seen on X-ray. Endoscopy—a procedure in which a tube is passed through the mouth or rectum—is needed to see these small, purplish lesions that lie just below the mucous-membrane surface. They can also be biopsied, but this is sometimes complicated by bleeding afterward.

In contrast to the treatment of infections, which is fairly standardized, the treatment of KS often varies from hospital to hospital. The reason for this is two fold. First, KS in the setting of AIDS is a new problem and it may take years to determine what treatment is best. For example, a drug that has the best results after six months may not protect patients from relapses as well as another drug that has less impressive results initially but offers better results two years later. Not enough time has elapsed to gather this long-term experience for AIDS patients with KS.

The second reason for variation in the treatment of KS in AIDS is that it presents a conceptual dilemma. KS is a cancer that appears related to impairment of the immune system. But many anticancer drugs suppress the immune system. Although these anticancer drugs may rid a patient of KS, they also tend to exacerbate the underlying immune problem. Patients become more vulnerable to opportunistic infections while they are being treated for cancer. While this is a risk for any cancer patient, AIDS patients have a very high mortality rate from these infections because their immune systems don't recover when the treatment is stopped. This dilemma has given rise to two approaches to treating KS in AIDS patients. Some investigators are using traditional anticancer drugs and radiation; others are using drugs meant to bolster the immune system, drugs known as "immunomodulators." It is too early to tell which approach offers better results. It may also turn out that one treatment works better with mild disease and another approach is more effective for advanced cases.

Standard Anticancer Treatment. Radiation therapy is effective for small, superficial skin lesions. For widespread disease, a combination of the anticancer drugs bleomycin, doxorubicin, and vinblastine is the most common treatment. Frequent side effects of these drugs are lung disease, allergic reactions, fever, hair loss, nausea, and vomiting from bleomycin; heart disease and hair loss from the doxorubicin; nerve damage that causes numbness and tingling in the hands and feet, and constipation from the vinblastine. A new drug that is used alone, called VP-16, is also being tried.

The Immunomodulators. The theory behind the use of these drugs is that boosting the immune system will cure KS and prevent opportunistic infections in the future.

INTERFERON. Although it has recently been discovered that there are three types of interferon, the classic interferon is a protein made by white blood cells that have been infected with a virus. This protein protects noninfected cells from infection. Interferon has been shown to have three effects: It has an antiviral action; it limits the spread of cancer; and it boosts the immune system in a general way. The main side effects of interferon injections are malaise, fever, and low white-blood-cell counts. Of the immunomodulators, interferon is the best-known and, for the moment, the most promising as a treatment for KS. It is extremely expensive and only available at certain hospitals.

THYMOSIN. This is a hormone-like substance that is derived from the thymus, the gland that influences the development of T lymphocytes. The side effects are minimal, usually a mild allergic reaction. This agent is being studied, but experience with it is very limited.

INTERLEUKIN-2. This is a substance made by T lymphocytes that stimulates helper-cell function. It is very difficult to produce in the laboratory, hence its use is currently impractical.

Lymphomas

Two rare lymphomas appear to be part of the spectrum of rare diseases seen in AIDS patients. As a rule, lymphomas are cancers that start in the lymph nodes and are cancers of the lymphocytes living within the nodes—in contrast to KS, which may start in the lymph node but is not a malignancy of white blood cells. The two rare lymphomas are Burkitt's lymphoma and diffuse undifferentiated non-Hodgkin's lymphoma (DUNHL).

Only one case of Burkitt's and no cases of DUNHL were reported among persons between the ages of 20 and 39 living in the San Francisco area between 1977 and 1980. But on June 4, 1982, the CDC reported four cases of DUNHL in the San Francisco area over a ten-month period; all four patients were young gay men. DUNHL tends to be a very widespread and rapidly advancing lymphoma. It may begin as a solitary tumor, but it usually spreads quickly to other organs.

Burkitt's lymphoma is rarely seen in the United States. It is, however, epidemic in parts of East Africa and New Guinea. The cancer has been strongly linked to infection with the Epstein-Barr virus. Classically, Burkitt's begins as a tumor in the jaw. A few cases have been seen in AIDS patients.

Both DUNHL and Burkitt's are diagnosed through biopsies. Although they are different diseases, they may be difficult to differentiate under the microscope. They are treated with anticancer drugs.

Gastrointestinal Cancer

Some investigators have reported higher rates of anal and oral cancers among gay men than in the general public. But the increased incidence seems to predate AIDS, suggesting that anal and oral cancers may be caused by local infection and trauma rather than by the immune suppression of AIDS.

A very rare form of colon cancer, called "cloacogenic cancer" because of the cell in which it starts, has been seen in AIDS patients. This is thought to be related to AIDS, but the limited number of cases make the association hard to prove.

GENERALIZED LYMPH-NODE SWELLING

On May 21, 1982, the CDC reported that generalized lymph-node swelling was being seen among gay men. What made this finding so worrisome was the knowledge that many AIDS patients had developed lymph-node enlargement before developing KS or PCP. While the syndrome seems clearly related to AIDS, no one knows what the relationship is.

A patient is considered to have the syndrome if he has enlarged lymph nodes in two separate areas (excluding the groin) for at least three months; if a node is biopsied and shows nonspecific changes; and if no other cause for the lymph-node swelling can be found.

AIDS is by no means the only or the most likely cause of such swelling. Infections such as hepatitis B, mononucleosis, CMV, tuberculosis, syphilis, and toxoplasmosis can cause it. Drugs such as heroin or Dilantin can do it. Cancers, particularly lymphomas and leukemias, can cause node enlargement. And autoimmune diseases, such as lupus, also cause lymph-node swelling. All of these must be excluded by appropriate tests before lymph-node enlargement can be called AIDS-related.

In the CDC report, there were 57 men who met the conditions of this syndrome; 86 percent were gay and 14 percent were bisexual. Seventy percent had constitutional symptoms that included fatigue, fever, night sweats, and weight loss. Most patients had enlargement of lymph nodes in the neck, armpits, and groin. On an average, the swelling had been present for 11 months. One-quarter of the patients also had enlargement of the liver and spleen. Some of the patients had the abnormal helper/suppressor T-cell ratio seen in AIDS. Three months after the study, one patient had developed KS.

The study was significant in light of past experience with AIDS. Of 73 patients with KS who were reported to the CDC between June 1981 and January 1982, 44 percent had a history of generalized lymph-node swelling before the diagnosis was known; of 61 patients with PCP, 23 percent had a similar history.

Generalized lymph-node swelling seems clearly related to AIDS. But it still isn't known whether this syndrome is a forerunner of AIDS or whether it is a milder version of the disease. Will patients go on to develop full-blown AIDS or will they be spared?

Men who have lymph-node swelling should see their doctors. It is important to exclude all the known causes. But for the time being, there is no treatment if it is AIDS-related.

AUTOIMMUNE DISEASES

There are many diseases that are classified as "autoimmune." Although they are highly varied in terms of symptoms, they share a common denominator: the body starts to attack itself, making antibodies against its own tissues.

An autoimmune disease in which antibodies are made against platelets—the blood cells needed for clotting—is thought to be part of AIDS. The disorder is called "idiopathic thrombocytopenic purpura"—ITP for short. Because of the decrease in platelets that results from these abnormal antibodies, patients may develop small purplish spots beneath the skin's surface and internal bleeding. Sometimes ITP doesn't cause any symptoms but is diagnosed simply because a low platelet count was noticed on a routine blood test.

One New York study reported that thirteen cases of ITP were seen in gay men after November 1980; two patients also had KS. This cluster of cases is very unusual since ITP is much more common in women than men. Another recent study reported a second unusual cluster in patients at risk for AIDS: five cases of ITP in hemophiliacs, all of them, also, male. Three of these patients had the abnormal helper/suppressor ratio that characterizes AIDS.

THE PSYCHOLOGICAL SIDE OF AIDS

Any life-threatening illness imposes enormous psychological stress, and AIDS is no exception. Patients, lovers, friends, and relatives suddenly have to face a potentially devastating disease.

No one adjusts easily to having a serious illness. But, as a general rule, patients who coped well with life before they got sick, who have a strong support network, and who have medical care that combines technical excellence with compassion fare better.

Even though people find different ways of coping, most people go through common stages before they finally come to terms with their illness. At first, there is a strong impulse to deny the diagnosis. But the denial has to be overcome in order to seek medical care. At this point most patients accept the reality, but not without anger and not without the question "Why me?" After one has lived with the diagnosis for a while, depression often sets in. The depression is compounded by feeling sick from the disease and from the medications. Patients get very depressed about changes in appearance, such as hair loss from the anticancer drugs. Following a period of depression, most people learn to cope.

Although people move through these stages of adjustment with some degree of predictability, emotional reactions can vary from moment to moment. There will be good and bad days, days when patients may want to talk about death and days when denial is a marvelous thing.

Certain specific tactics may help people cope. Patients often find it useful to talk to others with the same disease, to talk to people who know what it's like from the inside. Many people find that only those who have gone through a similar experience really understand what it's like. This doesn't mean that other people aren't supportive, kind, or needed; it simply means that they don't offer the same kind of understanding as other AIDS patients.

Patients may also find it helpful to talk with psychiatrists, psychotherapists, religious advisers, social workers, or anyone who has experience in helping people cope. It can be extremely useful to air one's thoughts and feelings to a neutral party, without the worry that one might be offending a friend or driving a lover away.

Coping with AIDS is also difficult for the visitors—the friends, lovers, and relatives. They can find rage directed at them or spend long hours sitting by someone's bedside in silence, feeling sad and powerless. Perhaps the most useful advice for the visitors is that they have to know their limits and limitations. There is no point in being in the room if one feels angry at having to be there. On the other hand, sitting in silence and holding a sleeping patient's hand may have all the point in the world. A problem that frequently arises is that visitors are often tempted to make the conversation cheerful. This is fine if the patient is cheerful. But to deny someone's sadness by imposing verbal cheer can be one of the most depressing experiences—it simply confirms the person's isolation.

Patients also need to be able to talk to the medical staff taking care of them. One of the problems with treating AIDS is that it often requires many different specialists, giving the impression that there is no one person to turn to. There should be one doctor who is the primary physician, whose job it is to coordinate the patient's care. It is also very important that all tests and procedures be explained beforehand; surprises should be kept to a minimum. People are less frightened if they know what to expect and why something is needed.

THE FINANCIAL COST OF AIDS

It may seem trivial to discuss the financial cost of AIDS after talking about the physical and emotional consequences, but the finances underscore just how serious AIDS is. According to an estimate in May 1982, the average hospital stay for an AIDS patient cost $64,000. The first 300 cases of AIDS cost $18 million in hospital expenses alone. And these figures don't begin to address the problem of how much money is being spent on research and how much more is needed.

PREVENTION

With any disease that is incurable and has such high stakes, the emphasis is on prevention. The best way to protect oneself is to limit the number of one's sexual partners and to know who they are. Having anonymous sexual partners is extremely dangerous when the risk of acquiring an STD includes the risk of catching AIDS.

Those who have AIDS, or AIDS-related symptoms, should seek prompt medical care since early treatment may improve the chances of survival. But people who think that they may have AIDS, or know that they do, must also try to protect others. This means not having sex with people without a full disclosure of the problem. It also means not donating blood.

Controlling AIDS has to be a cooperative venture.

HEPATITIS

Many things cause hepatitis and many groups of people get it. Infections, alcohol, and prescribed or illicit drugs can all cause hepatitis. Gay men, travelers, hemodialysis patients, drug addicts, and raw-shellfish eaters are some of the people who have a higher-than-average risk of getting hepatitis. But the term "hepatitis" only means inflammation of the liver—it says nothing about what caused the hepatitis or who got sick.

There are 55,000 cases of hepatitis reported to the CDC each year. But according to the CDC, this represents only 10 to 20 percent of the actual number of cases—the real total is 500,000 cases annually.

Over the past decade, gay men have accounted for an increasing number of these cases, and infections have become the major cause of hepatitis among gay men. The vast majority of these infections are sexually acquired. It is perhaps stating the obvious, but only hepatitis caused by infections can be transmitted; hepatitis caused by alcohol or by an adverse reaction to medication is not contagious.

While many infections can inflame the liver, not all of them start in the liver or primarily affect the liver. For example, cytomegalovirus and syphilis can cause hepatitis but neither starts in the liver nor causes hepatitis as the major problem. The three viruses that are known as the "hepatitis viruses," on the other hand, start to multiply within the liver cells and primarily cause symptoms that are due to liver inflammation.

These three are hepatitis A, hepatitis B, and hepatitis non-A/non-B. For the sake of completeness, all three will be discussed, but it should be emphasized that most gay men who get hepatitis get either type A or B. Although hepatitis A is a serious problem because of the number of men who get it, type B is ultimately of greater concern because it can cause chronic liver disease and because one can transmit it long after recovering from the acute bout of hepatitis.

Since each of the three viruses has distinctive features—such as a particular incubation period, mode of transmission, or means of prevention—they are discussed separately.

Hepatitis A.

While all three viruses are contagious, this is the one that used to be called "infectious hepatitis" because it is the one responsible for epidemic outbreaks in communities that share common water supplies or food sources. It is also the type caught by eating contaminated raw shellfish. Recently, it has also been shown to be a sexually transmitted disease common in the gay community.

This RNA virus is shed in feces and acquired by ingestion. The virus is transmitted by the fecal-oral route, meaning that someone must swallow food that has been contaminated with feces or ingest actual feces. In practical terms, people get hepatitis A from food handlers who don't wash their hands thoroughly, from contaminated water supplies and shellfish, and through oral-anal sexual contact. Anilingus and fellatio after rectal intercourse are the sexual practices most likely to transmit this infection. It should be added, however, that these sexual practices can only transmit infection if one partner is contagious and the other not already immune to the virus.

Anyone who has had hepatitis A before won't get it again. But someone who is exposed and susceptible to the virus will, if he is going to develop symptoms—usually develop them 21 to 35 days after contact, although the incubation period can vary from 14 to 45 days.

Unfortunately, hepatitis A is most contagious before symptoms appear. The highest levels of the virus are found in the stool two to three weeks before jaundice sets in; this is the point of maximum infectivity. The levels of virus then drop off sharply, so that by the time that eyes turn yellow, most people are no longer highly contagious. It is safest, however, to wait until three weeks after jaundice has appeared before resuming sexual activity, because studies show that a few people remain contagious for as long as three weeks after they have become clinically ill.

Of the three varieties of viral hepatitis, type A is the least harmful because it doesn't cause chronic liver disease and because, once the infection is over, the patient won't transmit it to anyone else. After the illness is over, the patient will again have a normal liver, he will not be able to pass the infection on to anyone else, and he will be immune to hepatitis A in the future. But this immunity is strictly limited to type A; it offers no protection whatsoever against the other varieties.

Hepatitis B

Gay men as a group have one of the highest rates of hepatitis B infection. In many American cities, between one-third and one-half of new infections occur in gay men. Studies show that between 50 and 75 percent of gay men have or have had hepatitis B.

Hepatitis B used to be called "serum hepatitis." It is caused by a DNA virus that is carried in most body fluids—blood, saliva, semen, urine, and tears—but infection is most likely to result from contact with infected blood or semen.

Transmission of hepatitis B occurs when infected blood, semen, or saliva enters the body of a susceptible person (someone who has never had a hepatitis B infection) through broken skin or across the mucous membranes of the rectum, mouth, or urethra. Because many body fluids can transmit the virus, there are many ways to catch hepatitis B. Blood transfusions, needles—including those used for acupuncture, tattoos, or ear piercing—objects such as toothbrushes, cups, or razors, and sex can all transmit hepatitis B.

The sexual practice most likely to transmit the infection is anal-receptive intercourse. But it is also felt that the insertive partner can acquire the infection during anal-genital intercourse and that deep kissing can spread disease as well. Although these specific practices spread the infection, one's overall risk of acquiring hepatitis B is most closely linked to one's number of nonsteady partners. This is why the risk of catching hepatitis B increases with age—an older man has had more opportunity to have more partners.

Someone who has never had hepatitis B, and is therefore susceptible to it, usually develops symptoms 90 days after exposure. But the incubation period can be as short as one week or as long as six months. And many people develop such mild infections that they never have symptoms.

The danger of hepatitis B isn't simply that it makes large numbers of people feel sick temporarily. The real problems with this virus are that, unlike hepatitis A, it can live in the body for years, remaining capable of infecting other people, and that it can cause permanent liver damage.

People who have part of the hepatitis B virus, the hepatitis B surface antigen, in their blood for more than six months are known as "chronic carriers." Some people remain carriers for life. In addition to the liver problems that carriers may develop, they can spread the infection to others. The fact that hepatitis B can be spread for years after someone recovers from the initial infection, makes the disease very difficult to control.

Compared to the general population, a very high proportion of gay men are chronic carriers. It is estimated that 5 to 10 percent of gay men are chronic carriers—a figure significantly higher than the national average of 0.1 percent.

Most people probably discover that they are chronic carriers through routine screening blood tests. They get a blood test for hepatitis B, not because they have symptoms but for other reasons—because they are having a routine physical exam or they're donating blood. Most carriers are not aware of having or having had hepatitis. They don't have symptoms of liver inflammation when they are diagnosed and the original bout of liver inflammation may have been so mild that it went unnoticed at the time.

Once somebody is diagnosed as being a carrier, the problem then becomes how to live a normal life without jeopardizing the health of others. In terms of sexual activity, the safest thing to do is to choose partners who are immune to hepatitis B—either because they have had the infection themselves or because they have received the hepatitis B vaccine, which has recently become available.

All carriers are not equally contagious. Some people may wish to find out how infectious they are. This can be done with further blood tests, but the results give only a general idea about infectivity and cannot prove that one isn't contagious at all.

Although the acute illness caused by hepatitis B may be more severe than that caused by type A (hepatitis B does cause sudden and fatal liver failure, but in less than 1 percent of patients), the acute illness is not usually the major worry. Most people who become infected with the virus never know it since only 25 percent of patients ever develop jaundice. The more serious problem with hepatitis B is that many people develop some form of permanent liver damage. While 90 to 95 percent of patients recover completely from hepatitis B, the remaining 5 to 10 percent develop chronic liver disease. Given that 200,000 Americans contract hepatitis B annually, this is an enormous problem.

Chronic carriers are most likely to be the ones who suffer permanent liver damage. Such damage can take many forms, which, in order of increasing severity, are chronic persistent hepatitis, chronic active hepatitis, cirrhosis, and cancer of the liver.

To distinguish between a case of lingering acute hepatitis and chronic disease, an arbitrary time limit of six months has been set; if after this period the patient still has evidence of liver disease, he is said to have chronic hepatitis.

Persons with chronic liver disease may have no symptoms; nonspecific symptoms, such as fatigue and loss of appetite; or specific problems, such as a bleeding disorder. The only real way to distinguish between the many forms of chronic hepatitis is to do a liver biopsy. The information gained by a biopsy is important because it will give the patient an idea of what his future course will be and because it will suggest whether the liver disease should be treated. For example, chronic persistent hepatitis doesn't get worse, but chronic active hepatitis, cirrhosis, and cancer do. Therefore, someone who has chronic persistent hepatitis can expect his liver function to be relatively stable—his liver disease won't get worse with time—but patients with the other diagnoses may suffer progressive liver damage.

Chronic hepatitis B carriers have a high incidence of chronic active hepatitis; one out of four develop it. Men who are chronic carriers are more likely than women to develop this problem, although the reason for this isn't known.

Patients who are chronic carriers and show cirrhosis on biopsy—which is scarring of the liver rather than inflammation—are at higher risk for liver cancer. In areas of the world where a high proportion of the population are chronic carriers, there is a high rate of liver cancer. In Africa and the Far East, where 10 to 25 percent of the population are chronic carriers, there are 150 cases of liver cancer annually per 100,000 persons; in the United States, where on an average only .1 percent of the population are carriers, there are one to three cases annually per 100,000 persons.

One of the major advantages of the newly marketed hepatitis B vaccine is that it seems to prevent one from becoming a chronic carrier and therefore should reduce the threat of chronic liver disease due to hepatitis B.

Hepatitis Non-A/Non-B

This type is probably caused by more than one virus, but nobody knows for sure since the virus or viruses have not been isolated. This type is now the main cause of hepatitis due to blood transfusions. A 1980 government report stated that hepatitis non-A/non-B seems to be more common among gay men than among the general population. But since studies of spouses do not prove that the virus can be sexually transmitted, it isn't clear why this should be so. Although this type of hepatitis has not been proven to be an STD, it would be premature to say that it isn't.

The three things that can be said with reasonable certainty about hepatitis non-A/non-B are that it is transmitted in blood; that, like hepatitis B, it can cause permanent liver damage; and that one can be a chronic carrier. Because there are no specific blood tests for the disease, further clarification is difficult. This form of hepatitis is a diagnosis of exclusion—it is the cause of hepatitis once every other known cause is excluded.

SYMPTOMS

Regardless of the cause of hepatitis—whether it be drugs, alcohol, or infection—the symptoms are basically the same, although they may vary in severity. It is said that hepatitis B causes more-severe symptoms than type A; but given that 50 percent of people with hepatitis B don't have any symptoms, this is not an accurate way of making the diagnosis.

Liver inflammation may be so mild that a person doesn't notice anything abnormal. The only way that hepatitis is diagnosed in this situation is by doing blood tests. If the blood tests demonstrate that the liver is inflamed, then the patient has hepatitis regardless of whether he has symptoms. If the tests are normal, even if the patient is a chronic carrier of the hepatitis B virus, he doesn't have the disease hepatitis.

Those suffering from hepatitis may initially have flu-like symptoms of fever, headache, and malaise. If the illness is due to hepatitis B, there may also be joint aches and swelling, and a rash that resembles hives. Loss of appetite, loss of taste for cigarettes or particular foods, nausea, and vomiting are common complaints. Some people develop itching. There may be abdominal discomfort near the right front edge of the rib cage, where the liver sits. Then the classical signs of hepatitis set in: a yellow tint to the eyes and skin, known as jaundice; dark tea-colored urine; and light chalk-colored stools.

DIAGNOSIS

There are two parts to diagnosing hepatitis: establishing that liver inflammation exists and finding out what caused the hepatitis.

ESTABLISHING THAT LIVER INFLAMMATION EXISTS

This is done by blood tests. Several enzymes contained in the liver are released into the bloodstream when the liver is inflamed. Low levels of these enzymes are normally found in the blood, but these levels rise significantly when one has hepatitis. Because these enzymes have cumbersome names, they are usually referred to by their initials: SGPT (serum glutamic-pyruvic transaminase), SGOT (serum glutamic-oxalacetic transaminase), LDH (lactic dehydrogenase), and alkaline phosphatase (which isn't known by its initials).

The levels of bilirubin, a blood pigment normally broken down by the liver, also rise during hepatitis. When the bilirubin level goes above a certain threshold, one becomes jaundiced.

The liver-enzyme and bilirubin tests are collectively known as "liver-function tests." How often these blood tests should be repeated during a bout of hepatitis is a matter of the individual physician's judgment. Most patients have normal tests within three months; and unless the patient has chronic hepatitis, he will have normal liver-function tests within six months.

Other blood tests may be ordered, not for the purpose of diagnosing hepatitis but to assess whether complications have developed and how severe they are. Some patients become anemic—a complete blood count reveals whether this has happened. Patients with severe liver injury may develop bleeding problems—the prothrombin time test discloses this. Patients who have a lot of nausea and vomiting may throw their blood chemistries out of whack—a test of serum electrolytes establishes whether this has happened. Patients with extensive liver damage may become confused and even stuporous—a variety of blood tests can be done to prove that this is due to liver malfunction, but if this complication develops, the patient needs to be hospitalized.

If the patient has normal liver-function tests and feels well by the end of six months, no further tests need be done unless he is a hepatitis B carrier. In this case, he should probably have an annual blood test to make sure that his liver continues to function normally.

The patient who still has high liver-function tests after six months, and therefore has chronic hepatitis, may need a liver biopsy to find out exactly what the state of the liver is. For this he needs to be hospitalized. Under local anesthesia, while he is lying in bed, a thin needle is quickly inserted into the liver and then withdrawn. The tissue is sent to the pathologist, the doctor who diagnoses what type of chronic liver disease the patient has, depending on what the biopsy specimen looks like under the microscope.

FINDING OUT WHAT CAUSED THE HEPATITIS

Once the diagnosis of hepatitis is made, the task is to find out what caused it. This not only helps the patient understand his disease but also helps him understand how to avoid giving it to others, and determines what, if any, preventive measures will benefit his sexual partners. In addition to the blood tests that differentiate between hepatitis A and B (remember that there are none for type non-A/non-B), the patient's history is very important. Patients should tell the doctor how much alcohol they drink, what drugs or medications they use, whether they have been exposed to anyone with hepatitis, whether they have eaten raw shellfish, whether they have traveled anywhere recently, and what their level of sexual activity has been. This information will help the doctor determine the cause of hepatitis.

Hepatitis A

The diagnosis is made by testing the blood for antibody to this virus. An "antibody" is what the body makes to defend itself against an "antigen"—something that the body's immune system perceives as a foreign substance. In this case the foreign substance, or antigen, is a virus. The body doesn't make an antibody to an infectious agent unless it has been exposed to it. The patient may not recall having had hepatitis, but finding the antibody in his blood proves that his body does remember. Having the antibody to a hepatitis virus is also what makes one immune to future infections from this virus.

Simply finding the antibody to type A doesn't distinguish between past and present infections, however. Someone may have had hepatitis A years ago, and now his hepatitis is caused by type B. The way to differentiate between former and current infections is to find out the class of antibody: is it IgG or IgM? IgG means that the patient had hepatitis A in the past; IgM means that he has it now, since the IgM antibody is present for only 45 to 60 days after the onset of infection. A fairly new test, the IgM radioimmunoassay, can now accurately diagnose acute hepatitis A.

Hepatitis B

The tests for this virus are far more elaborate because different parts of the virus can be considered as different antigens and each antigen has its own antibody. The tests for these antigens and antibodies each provide useful clinical information.

The Acute Episode. The first thing to test for is the hepatitis B surface antigen, which is part of the outer aspect of the virus. A patient with acute hepatitis who is surface-antigen-positive is usually assumed to have hepatitis B, although in fact he may be a carrier who now has hepatitis due to another virus. Although not always done, a check for the IgM antibody to type A can be done to make sure that hepatitis A isn't causing the current infection.

Not all patients who have hepatitis B have the surface antigen, however. Five percent of patients don't have it during the acute infection. But they will have an antibody to another antigen circulating in their blood—an antibody to the core antigen. While there is no point in checking for core antibody in someone who is surface-antigen-positive, it should be checked in someone who is suspected of having type B but is surface-antigen-negative. The other situation in which a person with hepatitis B doesn't have the surface antigen in his blood arises if he is not tested for it until several months after the acute infection. This occurs because his body has had enough time to rid itself of the virus.

Past Infection. Those who recover successfully from hepatitis B develop antibodies to the surface antigen. They are surface-antigen-negative and surface-antibody positive. The surface antibody makes them immune to future infections from hepatitis B and the absence of surface antigen indicates that they are unable to transmit the infection to other people.

The Carrier State. Patients who have the hepatitis B surface antigen in their blood on at least two occasions six months apart are carriers. (The terms "chronic carrier" and "carrier" are used interchangeably.) Six months is the length of time used to define the carrier state because studies show that 90 to 95 percent of hepatitis B patients are free of this antigen after six months. While all carriers are theoretically contagious, some are much more likely to be so. Tests for another antigen, the *e* antigen, and the antibody against it, are used to gauge the relative degree of infectivity. Those carriers who have the *e* antigen are probably very infectious; those with the *e* antibody are usually—but not always—noncontagious. Many gay men who are carriers are *e*-antigen-positive; in one study, 60 to 70 percent of the gay male carriers were *e*-antigen positive. The suspected reason for such high rates is the short time between infection and testing for the antigen—usually less than ten years. As time passes, *e*-antigen levels tend to fall and *e*-antibody levels rise.

Hepatitis Non-A/Non-B

If the tests for hepatitis A and hepatitis B are negative, if there is no other infectious cause of hepatitis, and if there is no reason for the patient to have alcohol or drug-induced hepatitis, then hepatitis non-A/non-B becomes the diagnosis. This means that the patient should not have IgM antibody to type A, B surface antigen, or antibody to the B core antigen.

TREATMENT

Depending on how severe the symptoms are, some people with hepatitis choose to stay in bed and others to go about their normal activities. Only 5 percent of patients need to be hospitalized. Of the 200,000 cases of hepatitis B annually, it is estimated that 10,000 are hospitalized. The only people who usually need hospital care are those who have severe nausea and therefore can't consume enough fluids or a minimum amount of food, and those whose liver inflammation is so severe that it is complicated by bleeding problems or poor mental function.

People with mild hepatitis don't require a special diet, although some people develop a natural aversion to fatty foods. Those who have such severe liver inflammation that they become confused and lethargic are put on a special low-protein diet in the hospital.

It is very important, however, that patients with hepatitis not drink alcohol and not take any medications without first consulting their doctor, because alcohol and many drugs are metabolized by the liver and may aggravate its already inflamed state.

Patients with chronic hepatitis may need special treatment, depending on what the liver biopsy shows and on how sick the patient feels. Those with severe liver inflammation may be treated with corticosteroids or immunosuppressive drugs, but several reports now suggest that these drugs may worsen the problem if the patient continues to have the hepatitis B surface antigen in his blood. Recent studies show that interferon, a natural substance made by the white blood cells to fight viral infections, may help patients with chronic hepatitis. But treatment is highly individualized in this situation and patients should discuss their case with their doctor.

PREVENTION

Prevention comes in many forms. There are general measures. Fellatio after anal intercourse and anilingus are high-risk practices for hepatitis A; anal-receptive intercourse is high-risk for hepatitis B. These sexual practices are high-risk for catching the infections for the person not already immune to the viruses and whose partner is contagious. If a man doesn't know the status of his partners, he may wish to find out whether he is still susceptible to hepatitis A and B. This will also provide the opportunity to find out if he is a carrier of type B.

People who have hepatitis should try not to spread the infection. Those with type A should wait until three weeks after they started to develop jaundice before resuming sexual activity. Those with hepatitis B should wait until they are surface-antigen-negative; if they are carriers, they should restrict their partners to people who are immune or wait until a susceptible partner is vaccinated against the disease. Since the hepatitis B vaccine takes several months before it is fully protective, this means waiting some additional time—a subject that will be discussed in the section on hepatitis B vaccine.

It is also wise to practice good general hygiene during the infectious period, with special attention to handwashing after going to the bathroom and before eating. It is safest not to share eating utensils with housemates during the infectious phase.

Specific preventive measures against hepatitis are gamma globulin shots and, now, the vaccine against hepatitis B. The gamma globulin shots provide what is known as "passive immunity"—they provide the antibodies against infection; the body doesn't have to make anything. But passive immunity is short-lived. Gamma globulin shots are for people who know that they have recently had sexual contact with someone who has hepatitis. The hepatitis B vaccine causes "active immunity"—it provides the antigen and the body makes its own antibodies. This provides much longer protection, but there is a time lag between getting the vaccine and being protected against infection.

Hepatitis A

A sexual or household contact who has been exposed to hepatitis A within the past two weeks should get a gamma globulin shot. If more than two weeks have passed, it's not worth getting the injection, because after this time one has either escaped infection or become infected. The gamma globulin may not prevent infection entirely but it will make the symptoms milder. The dose recommended by the United States Public Health Service is .02 mg/kg; this is usually rounded off to 2 milliliters for adults. If someone is reexposed to hepatitis A more than two months after he received the shot, he needs another dose. This form of gamma globulin is inexpensive; it costs roughly $5.

Hepatitis B

The type of gamma globulin used to prevent hepatitis B is different from that used against type A; it has much higher levels of antibody to the type B virus. Known as hepatitis B immune globulin (HBIG), it costs roughly $100. To be effective, it should be given within one week of exposure, and protection lasts from one to three months. Five milliliters should be given at the time of exposure, and this dose should be repeated one month later. Once again, it may only reduce the severity of symptoms rather than prevent disease entirely. Because the injections are so expensive, patients are often tested before the shots are given to see whether they are already immune to hepatitis B. There is no point in giving the shot to somebody who is already immune.

The Hepatitis B Vaccine

This vaccine is a recent breakthrough in medical care. Under development for many years, the vaccine was marketed by Merck, Sharp and Dohme in July 1982 under the trade name Heptavax-B. Because the hepatitis virus can't be grown in tissue cultures, the vaccine is much more difficult to make than other successful vaccines, such as those against polio or measles. The source of this vaccine is human blood taken from carriers of hepatitis B. It is the first vaccine made from human blood to be approved by the Food and Drug Administration. Because it takes 65 weeks to make and has to go through several elaborate processes, the vaccine is very expensive—roughly $100—and supplies are limited.

Gay men were instrumental in the development of this vaccine. Many of them contributed blood from which the vaccine was made, and two of the three trials to test the vaccine's effectiveness were conducted among gay men. The third trial was run among hospital employees, many of whom are also at high risk for hepatitis B.

The best time for a man to be vaccinated is shortly after he becomes sexually active, since he is least likely to have had hepatitis at this point.

The vaccination consists of three shots that contain inactivated viral particles; two doses are given one month apart and a booster dose is given six months after the initial injection. The vaccine works because it contains the hepatitis B surface antigen, which stimulates the production of antibodies against this part of the virus. Antibodies against the surface antigen make one immune to infection from hepatitis B. Roughly 95 percent of patients develop sufficient antibodies to the surface antigen to protect them from infection.

Since the vaccine is a recent development, it is too early to tell how long immunity will last, but three to five years is the current estimate. Booster shots may be needed after that. Among more than 200,000 persons vaccinated so far, few serious reactions have been reported. Soreness and redness at the site of injection have been the main complaints.

While a carrier or someone who has fully recovered from hepatitis

B won't be harmed by the vaccine, neither will he be helped. To learn whether an individual will benefit from the vaccine, he can be screened beforehand to see if he is still susceptible to the virus. Carriers will have the surface antigen, and those who are immune because of previous infection will have the surface antibody. Alternatively, patients can be screened by testing for the core antibody, since both groups will have it.

The recommendations about who should be screened before being vaccinated are based on cost-benefit analyses. Screening tests for susceptibility cost less than the vaccine, but their cost—particularly if multiplied by many patients—is not insignificant. Since a large proportion of people who are at high risk for hepatitis B won't benefit from the vaccine because they've already had the infection, people who belong to high-risk groups should be screened first. The principle is that screening high-risk populations saves money; screening low-risk populations does not. A gay man who has been sexually active with multiple partners should be screened before being vaccinated.

It takes several months before one is protected by the vaccine because it takes time for the body to develop the protective antibodies. Roughly 80 percent of those vaccinated will be protected after the second shot; the remaining 10 to 15 percent will be protected after the third. Someone who has just been exposed to hepatitis B needs the hepatitis B immune globulin to protect him during the time lag before the vaccine works. This won't interfere with the future effectiveness of the vaccine, but it has not been determined whether it is best to give both injections at the same time. There is also a possibility that the person will get hepatitis from the exposure, and therefore the vaccine won't work.

Because the hepatitis B vaccine is made from the blood of chronic carriers, and many of these people are in the high-risk category for AIDS, there has been considerable concern about whether the vaccine could transmit AIDS. The current feeling is that the vaccine cannot transmit AIDS. This is based on the finding that thousands of people have been vaccinated and there has not been a single case of vaccine-associated AIDS. The vaccine also goes through elaborate processes that inactivate all known viruses, and each lot of the vaccine is tested in primates—none of whom have developed a disease similar to AIDS. Some people remain worried about the safety of the vaccine, however, because they feel that it hasn't been available long enough to know for sure that it can't transmit AIDS. The CDC and most medical authorities currently recommend the vaccine for persons at high risk for hepatitis B.

Hepatitis non-A/non-B

Patients who are exposed to this variety of hepatitis are given the same gamma globulin shot that is used against type A, since it is inexpensive and has negligible side effects. Although treatment does no harm, it is unclear whether it really does much good.

GI BLUES: THE INTESTINAL INFECTIONS

Parasites—Amebas and Giardia
Bacteria—Shigella, Salmonella, and Campylobacter
Worms—Pinworms and Strongyloides

Fifteen years ago, if someone spoke about STDs and intestinal infections in the same sentence, it would have seemed a non sequitur. But in the intervening years, the connection has entered the realm of well-accepted fact.

Many intestinal infections, caused by a variety of organisms that include parasites, bacteria, and worms are prevalent in the gay community and are passed from person to person through sexual contact. Sex that involves oral-anal contact—either directly, through anilingus, or indirectly after hands or genitals come into contact with feces—is the major reason that all of these intestinal infections are STDs among gay men.

THE PARASITES—Amebas and Giardia

Amebas

Recognition of intestinal infections as sexually transmitted diseases probably began when amebas were first noted in a group of people who were assumed to be unlikely candidates for this "tropical" disease: New York men who had never traveled abroad.

In 1968, Dr. Harry Most cited three cases of amebiasis—the disease caused by amebas—among gay men who lived in New York. This observation remained fairly obscure until 1972 when another New York physician found amebiasis in a cluster of gay men who hadn't traveled abroad but who lived in one area of the city—Greenwich Village. Concerned that a common water supply might be the source of the outbreak, he had the New York City Health Department investigate the possibility. But the water got a clean bill of health. Over the next five years, the suspicion that sexual activity linked amebiasis to the gay community was confirmed. In 1976, when the New York City Bureau of Venereal Disease Control became the first agency in a large American city to diagnose and treat 14 different STDs, amebiasis still wasn't one of these. By 1977, however, amebiasis finally gained formal recognition as an STD.

Amebiasis is hardly an obscure disease; worldwide, it is estimated that 10 percent of the population has it. But it is traditionally a tropical disease, affecting poor people in Africa, Asia, and South America, or tourists returning from those parts of the world. Its occurrence in the urban centers of North America was considered a rarity.

While the prevalence of amebiasis is low in the United States as a whole (thought to be roughly 3 percent), it is much higher in some gay communities, where it is estimated to affect from 30 to 50 percent of the population.

The principal cause of amebiasis in gay men is *Entamoeba histolytica.* In a small proportion of cases, *Dientamoeba fragilis* also causes the illness. Other amebas, such as *Entamoeba coli* or *hartmanni,* are innocent bystanders that don't warrant treatment, but they are often a tip-off that the more worrisome amebas will be found if thoroughly searched for.

Amebas belong to a class of infecting organisms known as protozoa. They are tiny, one-celled animals that invade a host animal and feed off him, hence the term "parasite." Different parasites choose different parts of the body for home and diet. While a protozoan such as *Plasmodium malariae* invades red blood cells, causing malaria, amebas and *Giardia* (the other main protozoan STD) live in the gut.

What distinguishes an ameba from other protozoans are the "feet" that it uses for self-propulsion. The scientific name for these feet is "pseudopodia."

SYMPTOMS

Amebiasis causes a wide range of symptoms ranging from none to severe bloody diarrhea. Fifty percent of persons infected with amebas have no symptoms at all, although having none now is no guarantee that symptoms won't develop many years down the road. People who do have symptoms may have them on a steady, day-to-day basis or, more often, intermittently.

Since amebas take up residence in the large intestine, or colon, symptoms are those of colitis. In fact, amebiasis can mimic the mild cramps or bowel irregularities of functional bowel disease or the severe bloody diarrhea of ulcerative colitis. Both of these diseases, whose causes are unknown, should not be diagnosed until infections—including parasites—are excluded.

The people who develop symptoms from amebas do so because the amebas invade the bowel wall rather than remaining within the gut's hollow tubing. Patients notice a change in their bowel habits, usually developing frequent and loose bowel movements but occasionally becoming constipated instead. They get lower abdominal pain, a bloated feeling, have a lot of gas, and are nauseated. They may feel tired and lose weight. In severe cases, patients develop profuse diarrhea that contains blood and mucus.

Rarely, amebas invade the appendix, causing the standard symptoms of appendicitis—pain in the right lower abdomen; loss of appetite; nausea and vomiting.

These gastrointestinal symptoms are the main ones suffered by men with sexually acquired amebiasis. But in areas of the world where amebiasis is endemic, other problems arise from amebas migrating out of the gut, via the bloodstream, to distant parts of the body. While this can theoretically occur in sexually acquired amebiasis, most physicians have not seen it happen.

The common destinations for amebas that escape from the colon are the liver and lungs, where they cause amebic abscesses. Liver abscesses, which are more common in persons who lack symptoms of intestinal disease, cause fever and an enlarged and tender liver, with pain below the front right edge of the rib cage. Lung abscesses cause cough, chest pain, and fever.

There are many suggestions as to why infections outside the gut are extremely rare among gay men. These include: a better level of general health than that of indigent people in the tropics—making the Americans more resistant to infections in general; the possibility that the strains of amebas causing infection in the United States are less aggressive; and that a protein-rich diet, which is more likely in the U.S. than in the tropics, offers some protection against amebiasis.

TRANSMISSION

In order to get amebas, one usually has to swallow them. This is called a "fecal-oral" route of transmission. The new host usually develops symptoms two to four weeks after contact, although the range is anywhere from one to fourteen weeks.

In poor countries, amebas are usually acquired by drinking contaminated water or ingesting contaminated food. But gay men in the United States usually get amebiasis because of oral-anal sexual contact. Anilingus is the practice most likely to spread disease. In a study of 126 gay men, the 39 who had amebiasis all practiced anilingus. Of even greater significance, none of the 12 men who never engaged in anilingus had amebas. But any practice that involves oral exposure to feces can transmit amebas, and fellatio after anal intercourse is another likely way to get them. In group sex situations, this occurrence accounts for much of the disease spread.

Men who have no intestinal symptoms but are passing the ameba in its cyst form are the most likely to transmit the infection. The reason is twofold. First, they don't know that they are contagious; as asymptomatic carriers of amebas, they are unlikely to contact a doctor for diagnosis and treatment. Second, the ameba they excrete in its "cyst" form is very capable of living outside the body on inanimate objects and remaining infectious. At room temperature, cysts can survive on sheets, towels, and mattresses for a week. Unlike herpes and gonorrhea, amebas can be acquired from inanimate objects.

Persons with amebic dysentery are less likely to transmit the disease sexually. First, they are more likely to be diagnosed and treated simply because they feel sick. Second, they tend to excrete the parasite in another form, as a "trophozoite." In this guise, the ameba dies quickly after leaving the body.

Although oral-anal contact is the basic explanation of how amebiasis has become an STD, another mode of transmission has been reported that may be relevant in rare instances. Recently, 36 cases of amebiasis were reported from a chiropractic clinic that used enemas as therapy. Shared douching equipment is thus also a potential way to get amebas.

DIAGNOSIS

The method of diagnosing amebiasis leaves a lot to be desired; it is costly, unpleasant, and can be inaccurate. The best test uses a fresh, purged stool specimen. The patient has to go to a special parasitology laboratory, where, unless he is having active diarrhea, he will be given a strong saline laxative, such as Fleet's Phospho-Soda, to induce diarrhea. The fresh stool is then examined under the microscope within one hour, looking for amebas in both the cyst and trophozoite form.

The second-best test uses a fresh stool specimen not preceded by a cathartic. A stool specimen brought to the lab by the patient can be tested for amebas, but only in the cyst form. A rectal smear, using a cotton swab, can be done, but this only detects 20 percent of cases.

Some laboratories are now doing stool cultures for amebas if the purged stool is negative. Because a reliable growth medium has not yet been found, this test gives variable results.

Many substances suppress amebas, thereby causing the stool exam to be negative when it should be positive. Antibiotics, such as erythromycin, tetracycline, or the sulfonamides; laxatives or antacids that contain castor oil or magnesium hydroxide (milk of magnesia, Gelusil, or Mylanta); antidiarrheal medications with bismuth or kaolin (Pepto-Bismol or Kaopectate); barium (used for X-ray studies of the gastrointestinal tract); and enemas (tap-water, soap, or saline) all interfere with stool tests for amebas and should be avoided for two weeks prior to the examination.

Even when stool tests are done by experts, they can be misinterpreted. White blood cells, which may be present when the bowel is inflamed, can be mistaken for amebas; in this case the test would be positive when it shouldn't be. There can also be confusion about what kind of amebas are present; since only *E. histolytica* and *D. fragilis* must be treated, the distinction is critical.

One note of caution, however. As mentioned earlier, the amebas that cause disease and those that don't often go hand in hand.

Therefore, a patient found to have only a type that doesn't cause disease should be retested, because frequently he will be found to have *E. histolytica* or *D. fragilis* in subsequent samples.

When all is said and done, a purged-stool test for amebas is the best test available but it has many shortcomings. The problem is compounded by the fact that someone may shed the cysts only intermittently. Anyone suspected of having amebas, either because of his symptoms or because he has had contact with someone known to have amebas, should probably have three stool tests before accepting negative results at face value.

There are other tests for amebiasis. One is a rectal biopsy. Using a sigmoidoscope—a tube inserted into the rectum—a tiny piece of tissue is removed for examination under the microscope for trophozoites, the form of the ameba when it invades tissue. This test is appropriate for somebody who has symptoms of amebiasis but who has had several negative stool examinations.

Blood tests are also available but are only useful for diagnosing patients with severe symptoms or disease that has spread beyond the gut. These tests are also not particularly helpful in assessing the efficacy of treatment, since they may remain positive even after the patient is cured. The situation in which blood tests may be valuable is that of the person who, because he has bloody diarrhea, is thought to have ulcerative colitis. While the patient with ulcerative colitis may benefit significantly from steroids, the patient with amebic colitis can die from this treatment. So for a gay man who is suspected of having ulcerative colitis and whose stool tests don't reveal amebas, a blood test is an added safety precaution against receiving the wrong treatment.

TREATMENT

Not only does the diagnosis of amebiasis leave much to be desired, so does the treatment. For a start, no one really knows what the best treatment is. The drugs are expensive, require a prolonged course of therapy, and often have unpleasant side effects; and when all is said and done, only 60 to 70 percent will be cured—the rest will need to be re-treated at least once.

Although the medical literature advises treating only those patients with *E. histolytica* or *D. fragilis,* some doctors treat patients who have symptoms of amebiasis but whose stool tests show only other types of amebas. The rationale for this approach is that disease-causing and non-disease-causing amebas are frequently associated.

E. Histolytica—Asymptomatic Cyst Carrier

Diiodohydroxyquin. This drug, whose trade name is Panaquin, is the preferred treatment for the asymptomatic cyst carrier. The dose is one 650mg tablet three times a day for a full twenty days. Common side effects are limited to mild GI distress: nausea, heartburn, cramps, diarrhea, and anal itching. But serious side effects have been reported. If used repeatedly, it can cause an optic neuritis, an inflammation of the main nerve in the eye, which can lead to blindness. Panaquin can also cause a variety of rashes, including a serious one in patients who develop boils in response to iodines. The drug should not be taken by anyone allergic to iodine, nor by anyone with chronic liver disease.

Metronidazole. Better known under its trade name of Flagyl, this drug is used to treat asymptomatic cyst carriers although it is officially approved by the Food and Drug Administration only for the treatment of patients who are symptomatic. The dose is three 250mg tablets three times a day for five to ten days.

Absolutely no alcohol should be consumed during this period, because even the smallest amount can cause a violent reaction marked by vomiting, abdominal cramps, and shock. This reaction is similar to the one caused when people who take Antabuse, a drug designed to help overcome alcoholism, consume alcohol; the reaction is thus called an Antabuse-like reaction.

Other common side effects of Flagyl are a metallic taste, dark urine, fatigue, and depression. Some people also suffer headaches, nausea, vomiting, and fever.

One of the main concerns about Flagyl stems from the fact that it is carcinogenic in rodents and mutagenic in bacteria. No one has shown that there are any analogous effects when the drug is given to human adults, but the experience in the laboratory makes many people queasy about its use, particularly if an alternative exists. Another problem with Flagyl is the emergence of drug resistance; although this is not widespread, Flagyl-resistant amebas have been reported.

The one big advantage of Flagyl is that it will simultaneously eradicate giardiasis, the other main protozoan affliction of gay men. Since concomitant infections are relatively common, with as many as 10 percent of gay men suffering from both protozoans if they have one of them, the overlap provided by Flagyl may be quite useful.

Diloxanide Furoate. This drug, whose trade name is Furamide, is still an investigational drug that is available only through the Parasitic Diseases Division of the Centers for Disease Control in Atlanta, Georgia. The dose is 500mg three times a day for ten days. Its big plus is that it acts locally within the gut and isn't absorbed into the bloodstream. Because of this, side effects are limited to GI symptoms—bloating and increased gas. The minus side, also due to its restricted area of action, is that, unlike Flagyl or Panaquin, it has no value for symptomatic patients, whose amebas have begun to invade the bowel wall.

Paromomycin. The dose of this drug, whose trade name is Humatin, is calculated according to the patient's weight: 25 to 30mg per kilogram (2.2 pounds), divided into three doses and given for seven days. Unless the colon is damaged by colitis, this drug, too, is not absorbed from the gut into the bloodstream and is therefore quite safe. A minor disadvantage is that by killing some of the normal bacteria that live in the gut, it can leave a patient with temporary diarrhea after treatment is over. The drug is very expensive, roughly $45 for a week's supply.

E. Histolytica—Treating the Patient with Symptoms

Most patients with symptoms are treated with two drugs; one drug is intended to eradicate the amebas that have invaded the bowel wall, and the other to kill the ones living freely inside the gut. The standard recommendation is Flagyl, 750mg three times a day for five to ten days, and diiodohydroxyquin, 650mg three times a day for twenty days. Other combinations are used, but these are too numerous to mention since there is little agreement on what the second choice should be.

A one-drug alternative that is probably less effective than the combination therapy is Humatin, in the same dose used to treat the asymptomatic cyst carrier.

Treatment of severe intestinal disease or amebiasis that has spread beyond the gut needs to be determined by a specialist, although a combination of diiodohydroxyquin and Flagyl is still likely to be used.

Dientamoeba fragilis. Either diiodohydroxyquin, also 650mg, three times a day for twenty days or tetracycline, 500mg, four times a day for ten days is recommended.

AFTER TREATMENT

Patients should have stool tests—and probably two of them—two weeks after treatment to make sure they are cured. Since 30 to 40 percent of patients are not cured by the first course of treatment, this is particularly important. The reason for failure may be either that the drugs didn't work or that the patient became reinfected in the interim. (Being cured once offers no protection against subsequent infections.)

Some people may continue to have diarrhea or other symptoms after they are in fact cured. This may be a residual effect of the amebas having irritated the colon, a situation that has been dubbed "postamebic colitis." It may also result from the antibiotics (notably Flagyl and Humatin) having killed normal gut bacteria. Although these symptoms may persist for months, they usually go away without further treatment.

PREVENTION

Because 50 percent of men with amebas have no symptoms; because amebas can survive outside the body and remain infectious; because tests fail to detect every case; and because not all people who are treated are cured, amebiasis is difficult to control.

Some tactics help, however. Good general health and a high-protein diet appear at least to stave off some of the symptoms. Eating garlic and kelp are said to be beneficial, but this has not been confirmed in official medical circles.

Avoiding oral-anal contact with infected sexual partners is the crux of prevention. The individual who has amebas should avoid these practices until he knows that he is cured, and the individual who has been exposed to amebas should have himself tested. Once again, although anilingus and fellatio after anal intercourse spread the disease, they can only do so if one partner is infected to begin with.

Washing the anal and genital areas with soap and water before sex may avoid spreading the infection. Douching, however, is not recommended since it may bring amebas from the colon down to the external anal region—thereby increasing the likelihood of transmission.

A RETROSPECTIVE NOTE

Although in the current light of AIDS no one questions that the ante of STDs has been raised, on a minor scale this started with the advent of amebiasis in the 1970s. While antibiotics were available and the repercussions of the disease were unpleasant but not fatal, amebiasis became the first widespread STD in the gay community that was truly difficult to treat. The rise of hepatitis as an STD during the same period confirmed the impression that STDs can once again be a serious medical problem in the postantibiotic era.

Giardia

Giardiasis, the disease caused by *Giardia lamblia,* is the other protozoan affliction of gay men. Traditionally, this disease has been a major cause of traveler's diarrhea, particularly among persons returning from Latin America, Russia, India, and the Far East. Waterborne epidemics have also occurred locally in Colorado, Utah, New York, and New Hampshire where contaminated mountain streams have often been blamed for the infections. The other traditional setting for giardiasis has been the patient with certain types of immunodeficiency diseases, with either generally low levels of immunoglobulins or with a specific lack of the immunoglobulin IgA.

But during the period in which amebas emerged as a major cause of intestinal infections among gay men, rising numbers of giardial infections also became apparent. Studies on the prevalence of parasitic infections in gay men show giardiasis to be less common than amebiasis—roughly 18 percent infection rates as opposed to 30 percent. Unfortunately, both of these figures are probably underestimates since a very high percentage of protozoan infections go undiagnosed because they fail to cause symptoms.

What distinguishes *Giardia* is also its mode of locomotion; it uses "flagella" to get around (as opposed to the pseudopodia of amebas).

Under the microscope, this protozoan, *Giardia lamblia,* looks like a face with two large eyes.

SYMPTOMS

Like amebas, giardia causes a range of symptoms that vary from none to chronic intestinal disturbances. But the symptoms differ from those of amebiasis because this parasite colonizes the small, rather than large, intestine.

If symptoms occur, they usually start one to three weeks after exposure. The diarrhea of giardiasis, unlike that of amebiasis, doesn't contain blood or mucus and is frequently foul-smelling. In the first few days, the diarrhea may be watery and explosive, but it usually settles down to become loose, bulky stools on an intermittent basis. Nausea, cramps, and increased gas are also common.

Long-standing infections can interfere with the absorption of vital nutrients from the small intestine into the bloodstream, causing deficiencies of fat, carbohydrate, and vitamin B_{12}. *Giardia* can also cause lactose intolerance if it damages the bowel wall; the symptoms of this disorder are similar to those of giardiasis except that they are provoked by eating milk products. Unlike amebas, giardia does not cause disease outside the gut.

TRANSMISSION

Giardia is acquired in the same fashion as amebas: Feces containing the parasite are swallowed. Once again, anilingus and fellatio after anal intercourse are the ways in which giardiasis has become a sexually transmitted disease. The cyst form of *Giardia,* like that of amebas, can survive outside the body, permitting giardia to be acquired from inanimate objects as well.

DIAGNOSIS

The best way to diagnose giardiasis is by doing a stool examination. If a purged stool is used both amebas and giardia will be looked for in the same specimen. Repeat stool tests may be necessary for diagnosing giardiasis. One study reports that 76 percent of cases were diagnosed on the first try, 90 percent on the second, and 98 percent on the third. Some doctors suggest that stool test results may be improved by taking a very strong laxative, such as a bottle of magnesium citrate, then discarding the first three stool specimens and looking at the subsequent ones. This would theoretically provide a fresher sample of the small intestine's contents, but controlled studies haven't been done to verify this hypothesis. The list of substances that interfere with finding amebas on a stool test also applies to giardia. The patient can also bring a stool specimen to the lab, but this is not as good as a fresh or purged-stool test.

If stool tests fail to reveal *Giardia* but the doctor still feels that this is the likely cause of a patient's symptoms, more-elaborate tests can be done. Samples can be taken directly from the duodenum, which is a segment of the small intestine. This can be done either by endoscopy, in which the patient (after being mildly sedated) swallows a long tube through which fluid is extracted, or by having the patient swallow a gelatin capsule that is attached to a string and that picks up duodenal fluid. The latter test is called an Enterotest. However, both of these procedures are unpleasant and are usually used only as a last resort.

TREATMENT

Treating giardiasis is an easier proposition than treating amebiasis. The drugs have fewer side effects and are more effective. Since treating giardiasis is fairly easy, some doctors will treat it empirically. This means that if the patient has the symptoms but stool tests are negative, he will be given a trial of medication to see if treatment eradicates the symptoms.

Quinacrine hydrochloride. This medication, whose trade name is Atabrine, is the drug of choice. The dose is 100mg three times a day, taken after meals, for five to ten days. This cures giardiasis in 80 to 85 percent of cases. Serious side effects, which include yellow discoloration of the skin and a drug-induced psychosis, are more likely in someone receiving a prolonged course of the drug. Mild side effects that have been reported are dizziness, headache, and vomiting.

Flagyl. The dose for treating giardiasis is 250mg three times a day for five days, which is one-third the dose given for amebiasis. Thus Flagyl will cure a patient with both infections only if it is used in doses appropriate for the treatment of amebiasis.

Furazolidone. The trade name is Furoxone and the dose is 100mg four times a day for seven days. The main side effects are nausea and vomiting, and, like Flagyl, it can turn the urine dark.

AFTER TREATMENT

Test-of-cure stool examinations need to be done two weeks after completing treatment.

PREVENTION

The spread of giardiasis is somewhat easier to control than that of amebiasis because it is easier to cure, thus shrinking the pool of potentially infectious persons. The problem remains that many, if not most, individuals with *Giardia* have no symptoms and therefore won't be tested unless screening policies are established to detect those people at risk but without complaints.

Men who don't want to run the risk of catching giardiasis can choose to avoid oral-anal sexual contact and fellatio after rectal intercourse if they don't know whether or not their partners might be infectious. Those men who know they have giardiasis should "quarantine" their rectal area until they are cured. Once again, washing the anogenital area before sex may help avoid disease transmission.

BACTERIAL DIARRHEA

Diarrhea caused by disease-provoking bacteria is a common phenomenon in all walks of life. For gay men, however, these infections have joined the ranks of STDs simply because gay sex is more likely to involve fecal-oral contact. While the list of bacteria responsible for these infections continues to grow, only the three—*Shigella, Salmonella,* and *Campylobacter*—that cause the majority of cases will be discussed.

Shigella

Traditionally, *Shigella* has been regarded as a cause of diarrhea among children and travelers. That it has also become a significant cause of bacterial diarrhea among gay men is illustrated by figures from San Francisco. Between 1967 and 1977, the ratio of men to women, under the age of 50, who had *Shigella* infections changed from 1:1 to 10:1, and there was a sharp rise in the total number of cases. This is the same period during which San Francisco witnessed a rapid growth of its gay community.

The disease, shigellosis, is caused by a bacteria that is rod-shaped and pink (after being treated with a Gram stain) under the microscope. It causes disease by actually invading the bowel wall.

SYMPTOMS

Symptoms vary from nonexistent to a profuse, watery diarrhea that can be bloody. There may also be high fevers, severe abdominal pain, and muscle aches. The sudden onset of crampy diarrhea with fever within three days of an "at-risk" sexual exposure strongly suggests this disease. The patient who is very sick is apt to find himself going to the local emergency room and would be well advised to suggest the diagnosis of shigellosis if the doctor doesn't.

Shigella can also cause a much milder illness marked by occasional cramps and intermittent diarrhea or cause no symptoms at all, another instance of the asymptomatic carrier.

TRANSMISSION

As an STD, shigellosis is spread by fecal-oral exposure, either directly, through anilingus, or indirectly, through fellatio after anal intercourse. Nonsexually, shigellosis is most often spread by infected food handlers.

The incubation period is very short, usually from two to four days, but can vary from one to seven days. Shigellosis is an easy disease to catch because so few bacteria need to be ingested; it is estimated that 10 to 100 suffice. The other characteristic of the bacteria that facilitates its spread is that someone can be a carrier for a very long time—up to one year (although three months is more common).

DIAGNOSIS

Shigella is diagnosed by a stool culture taken with a cotton swab that is inserted into the rectum and then rubbed onto a special culture medium known as MacConkey's shigella-salmonella agar. As the name suggests, this is the same culture medium that is also used to diagnose *Salmonella*. Results take 24 to 48 hours.

TREATMENT

Drinking enough fluids to replace those lost by diarrhea is the core of treatment; antibiotics are secondary. The reason is that most patients with shigellosis get better by themselves within one week. Antibiotics may shorten the course of the illness and will prevent a relapse, which would otherwise occur in 10 percent of patients. But unless the patient is very ill, he shouldn't be treated with antibiotics until the culture report confirms that he has shigellosis. The patient with tolerable symptoms should also avoid taking antidiarrheal medications since these might prolong the course of the illness.

Since the asymptomatic *Shigella* carrier can spread the disease through sex, he, too, should be treated and his partners tested for the disease.

Several antibiotics, all of which have a low incidence of side effects, can be used to treat shigellosis. The problem is that many strains of the bacteria have developed resistance to them, particularly to ampicillin and to tetracycline. Patterns of antibiotic resistance vary from one geographic location to another. Therefore, if the infection is so severe that it needs to be treated immediately, the doctor should check what antibiotics the *Shigella* in the area have been sensitive to. If there isn't this time pressure, the doctor can wait for the culture report, which, in addition to confirming the diagnosis, will list the effective antibiotics.

Trimethoprim/Sulfamethoxazole. Better known by its trade names, Septra and Bactrim, this drug is a fixed combination of two antibiotics. The dose is one double-strength tablet twice a day for seven days. This is the drug of choice according to the Centers for Disease Control.

Ampicillin. The dose is 500mg four times a day for seven days. While amoxicillin can be used instead of ampicillin for treating many other infections, amoxicillin should not be used to treat shigellosis, according to the CDC.

Tetracycline. The dose is 500mg four times a day for seven days. Antacids and milk products interfere with the absorption of tetracycline, and so shouldn't be taken at the same time. The solution is to take tetracycline one hour before eating anything or two hours after eating.

PREVENTION

Careful handwashing and avoiding oral-anal contact are the measures to take for someone who is contagious. A person whose sexual partner has shigellosis should be tested and treated if he has acquired the infection. Again, washing the anogenital region with soap and water before sex may help prevent the spread of infection.

Salmonella

Salmonella intestinal infections are very similar to those caused by *Shigella*. Traditionally, *Salmonella* gastroenteritis is the result of eating contaminated food, especially contaminated poultry, but the prevalence of oral-fecal contact in gay sex has led to this disease becoming an STD for gay men although it is widely distributed in the general population. While it is certain that *Salmonella* can be sexually transmitted, it is not as well documented that salmonellosis, as an STD, poses as significant a problem for gay men as does shigellosis.

SYMPTOMS

Salmonella, whose appearance under the microscope resembles that of *Shigella,* causes GI symptoms that are virtually indistinguishable from those of shigellosis. *Salmonella* gastroenteritis is also a self-limited disease that usually goes away in two to five days, although it can last as long as two weeks.

However, if a large dose of a certain strain is ingested, *Salmonella* can cause another problem: typhoid fever. This illness is characterized by headache, fever, a transient rash, abdominal discomfort, an enlarged spleen, and a low white-blood-cell count. The vast majority of persons with sexually acquired *Salmonella* infections don't get typhoid fever, but sexually acquired typhoid fever has been known to occur.

TRANSMISSION

Oral-fecal contact is responsible for salmonellosis as an STD. The usual incubation period for the gastroenteritis is 12 to 36 hours, but symptoms can start anywhere from 6 to 72 hours after exposure. The incubation period for typhoid fever is longer; 10 days is average, but the span can range from 3 to 60 days.

Salmonellosis is harder to catch than shigellosis for two reasons. First, one needs to swallow a large number of bacteria, whereas very few shigella organisms will suffice. Secondly, the asymptomatic carrier state of salmonellosis is shorter than that of shigellosis, a fact that helps shrink the pool of potentially contagious persons. Even though salmonellosis is harder to catch, washing the anogenital region before sex may still be beneficial.

DIAGNOSIS

Stool cultures are the mainstay of diagnosis. The test is the same as that done for *Shigella,* and both bacteria will be looked for in the specimen.

The diagnosis of typhoid fever requires blood tests as well.

TREATMENT

Both the asymptomatic carrier and the patient whose symptoms aren't severe should not be treated. The reason is that antibiotics have been shown to prolong the carrier state—the period during which one remains contagious to others.

On the other hand, patients with typhoid fever do need antibiotics. The choices are:

Ampicillin. The dose is 100mg/kg, divided into four doses and given for fourteen days, or—

Chloramphenicol. The dose is 50mg/kg, divided into four doses and given for fourteen days. A severe anemia is a potentially serious side effect of this antibiotic, but some strains of *Salmonella* are resistant to ampicillin.

Campylobacter

Only recently has *Campylobacter* been found to be a common cause of bacterial diarrhea. But during the short interval since its recognition, it has also been found to be more common than either *Shigella* or *Salmonella* as a cause of bacterial diarrhea in adult Americans. While the bacteria can be sexually transmitted, it isn't known how often this occurs.

SYMPTOMS

The symptoms are the same as those caused by the other two bacteria and vary from mild to severe bloody diarrhea.

TRANSMISSION

Oral-fecal contact is again responsible. Because this bacterium has only recently received prominence, much less information is available about its incubation period, carrier state, or the ease of transmission.

DIAGNOSIS

Stool cultures are the tests that confirm the diagnosis, but not all laboratories have the special techniques required to culture *Campylobacter*. Recently, investigators from Oregon reported good results when they tried to diagnose this bacterium by another method. Using a Gram stain of a rectal smear, then examining it under the microscope, they found that the bacterium had a distinctive appearance. It was a Gram-negative bacterium that had "gull wings." If the Gram stain proves to be a reliable way of diagnosing *Campylobacter,* it would be an improvement over having to do a culture, because it is quicker and less expensive.

TREATMENT

Patients with symptoms caused by *Campylobacter* should be treated as soon as possible with erythromycin, 500mg four times a day for seven days.

WORMS—PINWORMS AND STRONGYLOIDES

The medical term for "worms" is "helminths." They are another variety of parasite. Unlike the one-celled protozoans that are also parasites, helminths are multicellular animals that may be large enough to see with the naked eye. Two types of helminths have been reported to be STDs in the gay community—pinworms and strongyloides. A brief discussion is included here for the sake of completeness; it is not meant to imply that helminths have become a widespread problem.

Pinworms

The technical name is *Enterobius vermicularis*. The female worm crawls outside the anus and lays her microscopic-sized eggs on the surrounding skin. Infection is acquired by swallowing the eggs. Since the eggs remain infectious outside the body, on sheets and towels, direct sexual contact is not a prerequisite of infection.

SYMPTOMS

The main symptom of pinworm infestation is rectal itching, which is usually worse at night.

DIAGNOSIS

The diagnosis is made by trapping the eggs on sticky cellophane tape and then looking for them under the microscope. The tape is wrapped around a flat stick, usually a tongue blade, and then applied to the perianal area. The patient can do this himself and then bring the specimen into the laboratory. Since it may take several attempts to capture the eggs, the test should be done on three to five consecutive days before it is called "negative."

TREATMENT

Mebendazole, whose trade name is Vermox, is the drug of choice. One 100mg tablet cures 90 percent of cases. Diarrhea and abdominal cramps are reported side effects, but these may be due to the expulsion of the pinworms rather than the drug.

Strongyloides

The full name of this helminth is *Strongyloides stercoralis.*

SYMPTOMS

It can cause intestinal disease, marked by abdominal pain, vomiting, and diarrhea or constipation. Strongyloides can also infect the lungs, in which case patients may develop a cough (sometimes coughing up blood) and shortness of breath.

DIAGNOSIS

A fresh stool specimen is examined under the microscope, looking for the helminth's larvae.

As a by-product of infection, patients may also have high levels of one type of white blood cell, the eosinophil. The combination of intestinal symptoms and high eosinophil levels should prompt a search for strongyloides.

TREATMENT

Thiabendazole (trade name Mintezol) in a dose of 25mg/kg is given twice a day for two consecutive days and should be taken after meals. Common side effects are nausea, vomiting, and dizziness.

AFTER TREATMENT

Three to four weeks after completing treatment, stools should be retested to make sure that the patient has been cured.

HERPES

The rising number of cases recognized during the past decade and the recent extensive press coverage of herpes, which has run the gamut from sensible to sensationalist, has made herpes a household word.

Herpes infections are not, in fact, new. Cold sores were described as early as 100 A.D., and genital herpes was described by the physician to the king of France in the eighteenth century. What is new is the rise in the number of cases seen by private physicians. In a study done by the Centers for Disease Control, there were nearly 30,000 such cases in 1966; by 1979 the number had risen to nearly 261,000. Since herpes is not a reportable disease—meaning that physicians are not obligated to report it to local health officials who in turn report it to the Centers for Disease Control—the true number of cases is not actually known. Current estimates are that 20 million Americans have herpes and that there are between 300,000 and 500,000 new cases each year. While most authorities agree that there is a "herpes epidemic," the lack of accurate statistics makes this impression hard to confirm.

Herpes simplex is the full name of this virus that is best known for causing cold sores or fever blisters and for causing the genital infections that are now attracting so much attention. Herpes varicella-zoster, a different virus that belongs to the same family, causes chicken pox and shingles, a disease in which blisters erupt along the path of a nerve root.

Herpes gets its name from the Greek word *herpein,* which means "to crawl." It belongs to a family of four DNA viruses that are collectively known as "herpesviruses." These four viruses share two distinctive features: mainly human beings are infected by them, and infection is not completely eradicated by the body's immune system; the virus lies dormant and may be reactivated many years after the initial infection.

Each virus causes a different clinical illness. Epstein-Barr virus causes mononucleosis and possibly cancer; cytomegalovirus causes a mononucleosis-like syndrome; and varicella-zoster (one virus that has two names) causes chicken pox and shingles. While the Epstein-Barr virus and cytomegalovirus lie dormant in white blood cells, varicella-zoster and herpes simplex lie dormant in nerve tissue.

In 1961 it was discovered that there are two sorts of herpes simplex: type 1 and type 2. Originally it was thought that type 1 caused cold sores (or infections above the waist) and that type 2 caused genital sores (or infections below the waist). While this is predominantly the case, the division is not absolute. Oral-genital and oral-anal sex probably explain why type 1 can be found below the waist, and type 2 above the waist.

In addition to the two types of herpes simplex, there are hundreds of thousands of strains of each variety. For the moment, the significance of this fact is unclear.

Genital herpes is primarily a disease of people in their twenties and thirties, presumably because they are the most active sexually. While nothing indicates that gay men suffer from it more than heterosexuals, particular problems that affect gay men—notably, rectal inflammation—have received less attention in the general press.

Although most cases of genital herpes are due to type 2, the initial symptoms are the same regardless of which virus is responsible. The percent of infections caused by each virus depends on the particular group being studied; it has been reported that type 1 causes anywhere from 10 to 40 percent of genital herpes infections. Interestingly, an individual who has already had a type 1 infection in the form of cold sores is much less likely to have a genital infection due to type 1 than someone who never had a cold sore. Thus, if a person has had fever blisters and then develops genital herpes, he probably has a type 2 infection.

Before describing the symptoms of herpes, a word of caution: not all people with herpes have symptoms. As with many other STDs, there seem to be some people who have the infection without having any physical signs of disease. These persons, known as asymptomatic carriers, can unknowingly infect their partners. While such carriers are one reason why certain STDs, such as hepatitis and gonorrhea, have spread so widely, it isn't really known whether this is a significant factor in the spread of herpes.

SYMPTOMS

The first attack of herpes is known as the "primary" infection. It usually occurs two to ten days after exposure to the virus through sexual contact. The classic symptoms are clusters of painful blisters or ulcers on the penis, near or in the rectum, or on the buttocks. The blisters may spread to the hands and thighs if the patient touches the original sores and then another part of his body. There may be itching or burning in the genital or rectal area, and the lymph nodes in the groin frequently become swollen.

About 10 percent of patients have infected throats, presumably from oral-genital sex. On rare occasions, herpes can cause urethritis, producing burning on urination and urinary frequency. It is estimated that 1 percent of nongonococcal urethritis is caused by herpes.

A particular problem that herpes can cause for gay men is rectal inflammation, also known as proctitis. The symptoms are severe rectal pain, itching, and diarrhea. Because the virus affects the nerves in this area, men may have difficulty starting the urinary stream, a sensation of not being able to empty the bladder, and have erectile problems. They may also be constipated and have weakness and pins-and-needles in the thighs. It isn't known how commonly herpes causes rectal inflammation, but one British study of 77 gay men with proctitis of unknown cause reported that herpes was responsible for 5 cases.

Besides these specific symptoms, 40 percent of patients with primary herpes have generalized constitutional symptoms—fever, muscle aches, and a vague feeling of being unwell. In addition, 4 to 8 percent of patients with primary herpes develop viral meningitis—an inflammation of the lining around the spinal cord and brain—due to herpes. They have a stiff neck, fever, severe headache, and vomiting. Although these patients should be hospitalized for proper diagnosis and care, they recover without complications.

This first attack of herpes tends to last longer and be more severe than subsequent attacks. Without any treatment, it usually takes two to three weeks to clear up, although it may take as long as six weeks. The blisters dry up, form scabs, and heal without leaving scars.

RECURRENT HERPES

Subsequent bouts are known as "recurrent" herpes. The virus, which lies dormant in the nerves near the base of the spine, becomes reactivated. While symptoms are similar to those seen in primary infections, they are usually milder and shorter-lived.

How often a person has recurrent attacks is unpredictable; some people never do, and others have frequent episodes. Some reports suggest that men are more likely than women to have recurrences; that those people who are prone to recurrences have an average of five to eight attacks a year; and that the frequency of recurrences diminishes over time. But these observations need to be taken with a grain of salt because they are not based on well-controlled scientific studies.

What does seem true is that patients with type 2 infections are more likely to have recurrences than those with type 1 infections. One study found that whereas 60 percent of patients with herpes 2 had recurrences, only 14 percent of those with herpes 1 experienced repeat attacks. The same researchers also found that patients with type 2 infections who developed high levels of "neutralizing" antibodies were more likely to have subsequent attacks than those with low antibody levels. It is unclear whether this means that a certain immune response predisposes someone to future attacks or simply that those with severe primary infections (and hence high antibody levels) are more apt to have recurrences.

Most people get a warning before the recurrent attack is about to start. They develop pain or itching in the buttock, genital area, or leg, starting anywhere from a few hours to a couple of days prior to the outbreak of blisters. It is important to recognize these warning signals, because this is the time to stop sexual contact in order to avoid spreading the infection.

What actually causes recurrences is unknown, but certain physical and psychological factors are thought to act as triggers. The list includes other illnesses, lack of sleep, exposure to sunlight, tight clothing, the physical trauma of sex, and emotional stress.

Some investigators think that not all "recurrences" are due to reactivation of the initial infection; they feel that people can be infected with different strains of the virus. This observation is controversial and most "recurrences" are probably genuine recurrences, meaning that they are due to reactivation of the original infection.

Again, the symptoms with recurrences are milder and shorter-lived than the initial bout. One-third of men have no pain with recurrent herpes; the only way they know that they are having an attack is by looking at their genitals. And recurrent attacks are usually over within ten days.

For many men, the major difficulty posed by recurrent herpes may be the psychological stress of coping with a chronic disease, a stress that has been reinforced by the press and solidified by the epithet "the herpes syndrome." While it is true that dealing with any problem that can't be cured is stressful, having herpes needn't engender a feeling of being a sexual outcast. Herpes may be a reminder that sex can have undesired aftereffects, but this message has been available to all sexually active people throughout the ages.

COMPLICATIONS

As with other sexually transmitted diseases, herpes also has some rare but serious complications. The virus can cause serious eye and brain infections, although these are usually caused by type 1 infections rather than by type 2. The eye infection tends to be caused by people touching their own blisters and then their eyes. It is painful and can cause blindness if not properly treated, but effective treatment is available. The brain infection, known as encephalitis, is much more serious. Unlike the meningitis, which is usually caused by the herpes 2 virus and which heals without complications, encephalitis is fatal in up to 80 percent of cases and often causes serious impairment even when it is treated promptly. Whereas meningitis causes a stiff neck and severe headache, encephalitis causes mental confusion, stupor, and seizures. Most patients with encephalitis do not seem to have had prior herpes blisters.

Another rare complication of herpes infections has been seen as part of the AID syndrome. Some AIDS sufferers have developed chronic herpes ulcers near the rectum. This complication has not been seen in gay men whose immune systems are functioning normally—but only in men who already had clear evidence of AIDS.

TRANSMISSION

Herpes requires close physical contact for spread; household contact is not sufficient. The virus is transmitted across the mucous membranes of the mouth, genitals, rectum, or eye. A recent report that herpes 2 could live outside the body—on toilet seats and towels for as long as three hours—caused alarm about possible new ways to catch the disease. But despite the fact that the virus may survive on inanimate objects, there is no proof that one can catch herpes this way.

Herpes is most contagious when someone has fluid-filled blisters. However, one should be considered potentially contagious from the moment warning signs start to the time that the blisters have healed completely and the skin looks normal once again.

Unfortunately, this strategy is not completely foolproof, because some people carry and shed the virus without having symptoms themselves. There is no solution to this problem since these persons are unlikely to know that they have the infection and certainly won't know when they are contagious. Fortunately, this is thought to be a rare way of acquiring herpes; most people get it from sexual contacts who have obvious signs of infection.

DIAGNOSIS

The diagnosis is often based on the history and physical examination rather than on laboratory testing. If the patient says that he has recurrent genital or rectal blisters that are painful, the diagnosis is usually presumed to be herpes.

However, patients may want to know with certainty what they have, and many doctors feel that the disease would be better understood if proof of the diagnosis were obtained. The best test for herpes is a viral culture. A cotton swab is applied to the fluid-filled blister and then sent to the laboratory in a transport medium. This test will also distinguish herpes 1 from herpes 2. Since not all laboratories are equipped to do viral cultures, the specimen may have to be sent to a specialized lab.

A quicker and less expensive test is the Tzanck preparation. The blister or ulcer is scraped—a procedure that is likely to be somewhat painful—and the material is put on a slide, stained, and then examined under the microscope. The test is positive if "giant cells" are seen; these are cells whose appearance has been altered by infection. However, this test is accurate in only 50 percent of cases: If giant cells are seen, the patient has herpes; but if not seen, the patient can still have herpes. The Tzanck preparation also cannot distinguish between herpes 1 and 2.

Blood tests for herpes are more problematic. While there are tests for antibodies to herpes simplex 1 and 2, these antibodies are so common that their presence can't be interpreted as proof that someone's current symptoms are due to herpes. At best, certain changes in antibody levels can be supporting evidence that symptoms were caused by herpes. If a patient has no antibodies during the initial attack and then develops them after the attack, or if the level after a recurrent attack is four times higher than before, this is a good indication that his symptoms were due to herpes. But there are many pitfalls to antibody testing: For example, patients with recurrent herpes often show no change in antibody levels before and after attacks, and 95 percent of the population have antibodies to herpes 1 before they ever become sexually active.

One of the difficulties with relying on the appearance of blisters to diagnose herpes is that other diseases may look similar. An unusual case of primary syphilis, with multiple painful blisters, can be confused with herpes, but a dark-field exam will readily make this diagnosis. Behçet's syndrome, a disease characterized by recurrent oral and genital ulcers whose cause is unknown, can also be confused with herpes. In the latter case, a negative herpes culture will differentiate the two.

TREATMENT

Primary Genital Herpes

With the recent release of the new antiviral drug acyclovir, specific treatment of genital herpes has finally become available. But because it is new, many questions are still being raised about its optimum use and potential shortcomings.

Acyclovir (trade name Zovirax) is effective against both herpes 1 and 2. Unlike many other antiviral medications, this one specifically attacks the virus and leaves normal cells alone; with many other drugs, it was a race to see whether the virus or the patient's cells would suffer first.

But acyclovir only stops the virus from multiplying. Unlike many antibiotics that are used to fight bacterial infections, which actually kill the bacteria, acyclovir doesn't kill the virus but only stunts its growth. This is why acyclovir can reduce symptoms and shorten the period during which one is contagious but doesn't actually cure herpes. And because acyclovir doesn't kill the virus, it can't prevent recurrences.

For persons whose immune systems are functioning normally, the Food and Drug Administration has approved acyclovir ointment only for the treatment of primary genital herpes. The drug was not approved for recurrent episodes because it has not been proven to provide significant clinical benefits. But the use of acyclovir for recurrent herpes is still a matter of scientific controversy, and studies are under way to try to settle the matter.

A practical dilemma faces patients and physicians about the use of acyclovir in recurrent episodes. Many patients will use it because nothing else helps (even though the acyclovir may not help either); and many doctors feel that if they refuse to prescribe it the patient will simply find another doctor who will. The reason for concern about misuse of the drug is the fear that the virus will become increasingly resistant to acyclovir. While this is not yet a widespread problem, cases have already been reported of herpes infections that are resistant to acyclovir.

To use acyclovir ointment correctly, it should be applied to all lesions as soon as possible after the symptoms of primary herpes start. The medication should be applied six times a day—this means every three hours while awake—for seven days. A rubber glove should be used to prevent spreading the infection to other parts of the body.

Nearly 30 percent of patients report a burning or stinging sensation when they apply acyclovir, but this is not an adverse reaction to the medication; it is only the transient effect of applying an ointment to lesions that are already sore.

Even though acyclovir is helpful, patients should remember that it is not a panacea. The drug has been shown to lessen the formation of new blisters and to shorten the period of symptoms and viral shedding during the initial attack—but only by approximately three days. And although it decreases the period of viral shedding during subsequent attacks, it has not been shown to have any significant effect on symptoms.

Since acyclovir ointment is not a perfect solution to the problem of genital herpes infections, other treatments are being investigated. These include other forms of acyclovir, such as the oral and intravenous preparations. There is some evidence that oral acyclovir may be more effective than the ointment for primary attacks, but this form of the drug has not yet been approved. The intravenous form of the drug was approved by the FDA in November 1982 for treatment of severe initial attacks of genital herpes in patients with normal immune systems and for treatment of initial and recurrent bouts of genital and oral herpes in immune-compromised patients. Most patients currently using acyclovir for genital herpes use the ointment.

Other alternatives are also being studied. Gossypol, a cottonseed-oil extract that is used as a male contraceptive in China, was recently found to kill the herpes virus in a laboratory setting. However, many substances have seemed useful in a test tube but have not turned out to be beneficial in patients. It is too early to tell whether gossypol will fall into this category.

Interferon, a natural substance made by the body's white blood cells, and vaccines against herpes 1 and 2 are also being investigated. But for the time being, there is no cure for genital herpes. Although a solution is being sought through a variety of approaches, there is no cure at present.

Recurrent Genital Herpes

Treatment basically involves good hygiene rather than medication. The lesions should be washed with soap and water and exposed to air for drying, rather than drying them with a towel. Anesthetic and antibiotic creams should be avoided.

Eye and Brain Infections

These rare and serious complications require specialized and individualized treatment. Eye infections are treated with ophthalmic drops that contain antiviral agents such as trifluorothymidine, idoxuridine, or adenine arabinoside. Brain infections are treated with intravenous adenine arabinoside.

PREVENTION

Avoiding direct sexual contact with someone who has active lesions is the best prevention. While it is possible to get herpes from someone who has the virus but doesn't have symptoms, most people acquire herpes from partners who do have visible lesions.

THE CLASSICS: SYPHILIS and GONORRHEA

New Variations on Old Themes

Syphilis and gonorrhea are the two diseases that spring to mind when people think of VD. While no one would dispute their significance, especially in the preantibiotic era, some might say that their importance has waned relative to today's gamut of sexually transmitted diseases.

It isn't a question of numbers; although it is true that syphilis is much less common today than it was 40 years ago, the incidence of gonorrhea has tripled in the same time period. Rather, it is that syphilis and gonorrhea, unlike many STDs today, can be easily diagnosed and cured.

Because there are screening tests for syphilis and gonorrhea, these infections can be detected before symptoms develop, before the person actually becomes ill. And because they are both bacterial diseases—unlike herpes and hepatitis, which are viral—they are readily cured by antibiotics. Since penicillin is the preferred antibiotic in most cases, the cure is low-cost and usually has no serious side effects. If promptly treated, syphilis and gonorrhea rarely cause long-term problems for men (although this isn't true for women, who can be quickly sterilized by unsuspected gonococcal infections that scar their fallopian tubes).

Even though syphilis and gonorrhea are easy to treat, prevention remains preferable to cure. But compared to many other STDs, which are either incurable or difficult to treat, syphilis and gonorrhea at least have the potential for being eradicated. It would be presumptuous to say that syphilis and gonorrhea are under control, but at least the technology is there.

Because of a tendency to lump the two diseases together, the descriptions that follow will highlight some of their differences.

Syphilis

Syphilis has long enjoyed the limelight of the venereal stage. Although some investigators detect references to it in the writings of the Greek physician Hippocrates, the first clear description comes from reports of the "great pox" (as distinct from "small") that swept across Europe and Asia in the fifteenth century. Colloquially, it is sometimes known as "bad blood" or "the syph."

The discovery of the spiral-shaped bacteria that causes it, *Treponema pallidum,* came five centuries later, in 1905. While the bacterium, also known as a spirochete, can be seen and grown in animals, it cannot be grown in normal laboratory cultures—a difficulty that has hampered research and the development of a vaccine.

Syphilis now ranks third—after gonorrhea and chickenpox—in the list of infectious diseases that health officials are obligated to report to the Centers for Disease Control in Atlanta, Georgia. There are roughly 30,000 new cases reported each year. If preexisting cases are counted, there are approximately 60,000 reported cases in the United States today. But the CDC estimates that for each reported case, there are three unreported ones. While the total number of cases today is much less than World War II levels, there is evidence that the downward trend is being reversed. The incidence of primary and secondary syphilis increased by more than 40 percent between 1978 and 1981.

Men represent a growing proportion of these cases. In 1950 the male-to-female ratio was roughly 1:1; by 1975 it was 2:1. Gay and bisexual men now account for 50 percent of new cases.

Syphilis is a disease that can be caught before or after birth. If someone gets syphilis while still in the womb, he has "congenital syphilis"; after that, he has "acquired syphilis." Since adults can get only acquired syphilis, the following discussion is exclusively about acquired syphilis.

SYMPTOMS

The symptoms of syphilis depend on how long one has had the infection. Each set period of time, with its distinctive symptoms, is known as a "stage." Not only are the symptoms of each stage different, but

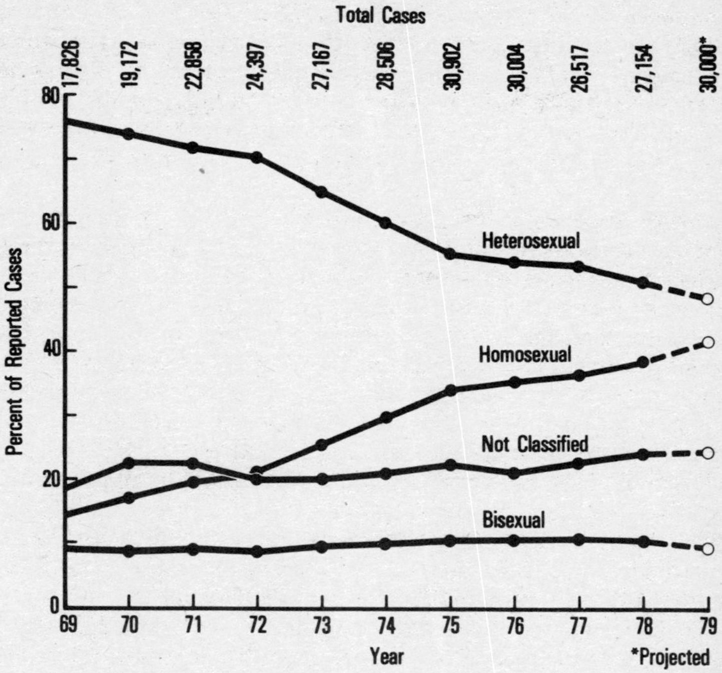

Sexually transmitted diseases, 1980 Status Report, NIAID Study Group

Source: U.S. Department of Health and Human Services, Public Health Service, Centers for Disease Control

the stage also determines how the disease should be diagnosed and treated.

The six stages of syphilis are grouped into the early stages and the late stages; the four early stages occur within the first year of infection and the two late stages occur any time after that. Early syphilis is much more common than late syphilis.

The Early Stages

Incubating Syphilis. This is the period after someone has come into contact with syphilis but before he has had time to develop the symptoms of primary syphilis. By definition, there are no symptoms during the incubating stage. The only way to suspect that a person has the infection is to know that he has had sexual contact with someone who has syphilis. The diagnosis may be hard to prove since many patients have negative blood tests for syphilis at this stage. Anyone with a partner during the past three months who had syphilis should be treated with antibiotics.

Primary Syphilis. Symptoms usually start two to four weeks after exposure, but the time lag can range from one week to three months. A person who has been exposed to many bacteria because his partner had a large open sore is likely to develop symptoms sooner than someone who was only exposed to a few bacteria because his partner's lesions were almost healed. The hallmark of primary syphilis is the "chancre." Classically, it is a single painless ulcer with raised firm borders that appears at the site of sexual contact: mouth, genitals, rectum, or perianal area. There is also painless swelling of the nearby lymph glands. Because 50 percent of chancres in gay men are rectal and because they are usually painless, the diagnosis of primary syphilis can be easily missed unless an adequate rectal exam is done.

Studies report, however, that less than half of all patients show the "classic" symptoms of textbook syphilis. Some people have multiple chancres that become painful because of abrasions or infection. Doctors can mistake these sores for herpes, chancroid, or granuloma inguinale (other STDs) or lichen planus (a skin disease). Rectal syphilis can also cause pain and discharge that may be confused with other causes of rectal inflammation, such as gonorrhea.

The chancre usually disappears in two to six weeks, but the lymph-node swelling can persist for months. The symptoms of primary syphilis eventually go away, whether or not the infection is treated.

Secondary Syphilis. If the primary stage is not treated, secondary syphilis usually develops six to eight weeks after the chancre heals—although it can take as long as six months to appear. Classically, primary syphilis is gone by the time secondary syphilis appears, but as many as one-third of patients still have a chancre when the symptoms of secondary syphilis develop.

Whereas primary syphilis is a localized disease, secondary is a generalized illness. A flu-like feeling with muscle and joint aches, fever, loss of appetite, weight loss, headache, and sore throat is common. Seventy percent of patients get a rash. Classically, the rash affects the palms and soles (places where very few rashes are found), occurs diffusely over the body, and affects the right and left sides of the body symmetrically. Anyone with this sort of rash should probably get a blood test for syphilis. Although it is said that the rash doesn't itch, recent studies suggest that in fact many patients do develop itching. The rash may also be so faint that it goes unnoticed.

Two other kinds of rashes typically occur in secondary syphilis. The first is called "condylomata lata." These large, wart-like lesions have a smooth surface and vary in color from grayish-white to pink or red. They occur in moist body folds—between the buttocks, in the perianal area, the inside of the upper thigh region, near the scrotum, in the armpits, and between the fingers and toes—and are extremely contagious. The other rash, called "mucous patches," consists of silvery-gray erosions on the mucous membranes of the mouth and genitalia.

Half of the patients with secondary syphilis get generalized lymph-node swelling that affects any of the nodes under the chin, behind the ears, in the neck, in the armpits, in the groin, or near the elbows. Unless the cause is known, a blood test for syphilis should be part of any evaluation of generalized lymph-node swelling.

Although a flu-like feeling, rash, and lymph-node swelling are the most common signs of secondary syphilis, this stage of the disease can affect many other organs. If the liver is affected, patients get the symptoms of hepatitis—abdominal discomfort, nausea, and loss of appetite. If the eye is involved, patients develop eye pain and visual difficulties. When the lining around the brain and spinal cord is affected, patients get headaches and stiff necks. Hair roots can also be affected by secondary syphilis, causing an increase in normal hair loss or patchy areas of baldness.

Just like primary syphilis, the symptoms of secondary syphilis go away whether or not the disease is treated.

Early Latent. This is the last of the "early" stages of syphilis; it is the period of time between the disappearance of the symptoms of secondary syphilis and the end of the first year of infection. Although there are no symptoms during this stage, there may be relapses of secondary syphilis—in which case the individual has secondary syphilis rather than early latent.

The Late Stages

Late Latent. During this phase, which occurs anytime after the first year, there are no symptoms and no relapses of secondary syphilis. And finally, most patients are no longer contagious.

Tertiary. Even without treatment, only 30 to 50 percent of patients would develop this stage, which can occur many years after the initial infection. Since the advent of penicillin, it has become extremely rare to see symptoms of tertiary syphilis.

There are three types of problems associated with this stage: "gummas," which are firm lesions that can occur in the skin, mucous membranes, hard palate, tongue, nasal septum, bones, muscles, and internal organs; "cardiovascular syphilis," and "neurosyphilis."

Cardiovascular syphilis, which affects the heart and blood vessels, is more common in blacks than whites. Nationally there are about 200 cases a year. It can cause enlargement of the aorta, the major artery that leads blood out of the heart and into the rest of the body; eventually this enlargement can cause a fatal rupture of the aorta. Cardiovascular syphilis can also cause the aortic valve, which regulates blood flow from the heart into the artery, to malfunction and can even cause an obstruction of the coronary arteries, which would simulate a heart attack.

Neurosyphilis, unlike the heart disease, is commoner in whites than blacks. There are roughly 100 cases a year. When it affects brain tissue, it causes a condition known as "general paresis of the insane." Patients gradually develop memory loss, poor judgment, speech problems, and loss of motor coordination. When it affects the nerve tissue of the spinal column, it is known as "tabes dorsalis"; patients develop shooting pains or numbness and tingling in the legs, impotence, and bowel and bladder problems. Neurosyphilis can also destroy joints by ruining the nerves that tell a joint when to stop bending; this is the "Charcot joint."

But neurosyphilis may not cause any symptoms. This is why some doctors recommend a spinal tap—the test needed to diagnose neurosyphilis—for anyone who has had syphilis for more than one year.

Other doctors may simply prescribe enough penicillin to treat neurosyphilis just in case the patient has it.

Fortunately, these myriad signs of syphilis, which earned it the title "the great imitator," are now extremely rare.

TRANSMISSION

In 95 percent of cases, syphilis is a sexually transmitted disease. The spirochete enters the body through broken skin or unbroken mucous membranes. Syphilis is extremely contagious through sexual contact during the primary and secondary stages—50 percent of contacts will become infected. It may also be contagious during the early latent stage, but this is probably due to relapses of secondary syphilis that go unnoticed. The disease can also be acquired nonsexually, through blood transfusions. Since blood is routinely checked for syphilis prior to transfusion, this is now a very rare occurrence. Because people with syphilis can have negative screening tests, however, this mode of transmission remains theoretically possible.

DIAGNOSIS

Syphilis can be diagnosed both in patients who have symptoms and in those who don't. Patients who are symptom-free can be diagnosed by blood tests. But much of the routine screening for syphilis is done because it is required by law for a marriage license. Unfortunately, gay men slip through this safety net thrown out for the heterosexual community. Since 50 percent of new infections now occur among gay men, much of the syphilis screening mandated by law is wasteful, because it leaves out many who are at high risk.

Blood Tests

Blood tests are the mainstay of screening patients without symptoms, for diagnosing patients with symptoms, and for checking that treatment has been adequate. There are two categories of blood tests: the nonspecific and the specific. Nonspecific tests, namely the VDRL (Venereal Disease Research Laboratory) and RPR (Rapid Plasma Reagin), are used for screening; they are called "nonspecific" because they detect a product resulting from the effect of the spirochete on the patient's cells rather than a specific antibody against the bacterium. Specific tests detect antibodies made against *T. pallidum.*

It is important to understand the meaning of test results to see how mistakes in diagnosis can arise and to know how test results should change after treatment.

The nonspecific tests—namely the RPR and the VDRL—are the screening tests, the ones used to detect syphilis in patients without symptoms. The RPR is often done in the doctor's office; the VDRL is usually done when blood is sent to the laboratory. Overall, the VDRL is probably the more common test. Although the results of both tests change after someone is treated, the VDRL is the one used to monitor the effectiveness of treatment.

Even when the tests are accurate (remembering that a laboratory can always make a mistake), their meaning can be misinterpreted. The first situation in which misinterpretation is likely to occur is in the person who has incubating syphilis, but still has a negative VDRL. This is because it takes time for the test to become positive—usually four to eight weeks after contact with the infection, or within two weeks of the chancre; thus a negative blood test two days after exposure is no guarantee that someone is disease-free. A person with tertiary syphilis may also have a negative VDRL, because his antibody response has died down.

These examples, which are "false negatives," illustrate situations in which someone can have syphilis and yet have a negative blood test, but the opposite problem can also arise—a person without syphilis can have a positive blood test. This is called a "false positive" reaction. This situation usually occurs in someone with a recent bacterial or viral infection, someone who has recently been vaccinated, someone who is elderly or a drug addict, or someone with an autoimmune disease such as systemic lupus erythematosus.

To avoid these mistakes in interpretation, the VDRL should be repeated about eight weeks after exposure if the patient's initial test was negative and he is thought to have incubating syphilis. If a person is suspected of having tertiary syphilis—if, for example, he remembers having a chancre many years ago but was never treated—he should have a specific test for syphilis. And anyone who has a positive VDRL or RPR should have a specific test for syphilis; if the specific test is negative, then he has a false positive VDRL or RPR and does not have syphilis.

Differentiating early latent from late latent syphilis may be difficult, but the distinction is important because the two stages are treated differently. A symptom-free person with a true positive VDRL has early latent syphilis if during the past year he had a negative VDRL, had symptoms that suggested primary or secondary syphilis, had sex with someone who had early syphilis, or if his VDRL antibody level has increased fourfold over the year. If none of these criteria is met, the patient is presumed to have late latent syphilis.

A word of caution about blindly relying on tests. The patient who looks as if he has redeveloped the signs of syphilis should be retreated regardless of what the blood test shows. And while most patients with secondary syphilis have very high antibody levels, 1 to 2 percent have a negative VDRL because of an unusual phenomenon known as the "prozone reaction." In this situation the test is negative if done on undiluted serum (the usual way to do it) but positive on a diluted specimen. It takes a special request from the doctor to repeat it this way.

As mentioned earlier, the VDRL is used not only to diagnose the disease but also to assess the effectiveness of treatment. This is done by looking at the amount of antibody detected by the VDRL; this amount is called the "titer." Whenever VDRL results are positive, they are quantified by titer (1:2, 1:4, 1:8, 1:16 . . . 1:256, etc.). A titer of 1:256 indicates many more antibodies than a titer of only 1:2. A negative VDRL means that there is no antibody. Treatment should lower the antibody level. Most patients who are treated for primary syphilis can expect their VDRLs to revert to negative within a year; those with secondary syphilis can expect the VDRL to become negative within two years; but those with late syphilis may have positive VDRLs for life even though they've been adequately treated. To make sure that treatment has been adequate, the VDRL should be repeated at three, six, and twelve months (and at twenty-four months for someone with secondary syphilis). If the VDRL increases fourfold (i.e., 1:16 to 1:256) or fails to drop fourfold from an initially high titer, re-treatment is necessary.

The specific blood tests for syphilis detect antibody to the spirochete. Although false positive results can occur, they are extremely rare. These tests are not used for screening purposes, nor are they used to see whether treatment is adequate. They are used to confirm the diagnosis of syphilis that is suspected on the basis of a positive VDRL or RPR.

The most widely used specific test is the FTA-ABS (fluorescent treponemal antibody-absorption). This test remains positive for life in those who have had syphilis, regardless of whether they have been treated. The FTA is reported as borderline, 1+, 2+, 3+, 4+. A borderline result should be repeated; if borderline twice, it is interpreted as positive.

Tests for the Spirochete

In addition to the blood tests, patients who have the chancres of primary syphilis or the condylomata lata of secondary syphilis should have samples scraped from these lesions and looked at under the microscope. Because the spirochete is too thin to be seen with the usual light microscope, it requires a special technique known as the "dark-field" exam. A positive test means that spirochetes were seen. Unless the specimen was taken from the mouth, where there are other spirochetes that look like *T. pallidum,* a positive dark-field exam provides unequivocal confirmation of syphilis. A negative test, however, doesn't mean that the person tested is disease-free, because a minimum number of bacteria must be present before they become visible. If the scraping was taken from a healing chancre, there may have been too few bacteria to see. The test should be repeated on three consecutive days before it is finally called "negative." Antiseptics applied to the skin lesions before scraping will also cause artificially negative results and so should not be used prior to testing.

NEUROSYPHILIS— A SPECIAL WORD ABOUT DIAGNOSIS

Neurosyphilis can be diagnosed only by doing a spinal tap. This procedure, which can be done in the doctor's office, involves inserting a needle into the middle of the low back, after the skin has been numbed, and withdrawing some fluid. In neurosyphilis the spinal fluid has a positive VDRL and some other nonspecific abnormalities. Theoretically, anyone who may have had syphilis for more than a year should have a spinal tap. But in practice, this is rarely done if patients don't have symptoms of neurosyphilis. Instead, patients are given enough penicillin to cure neurosyphilis should they have it. The potential problem with this strategy is that patients are treated with intramuscular injections of penicillin rather than the intravenous form of the antibiotic, which is used if someone is known to have neurosyphilis; and intramuscular penicillin may not be as effective.

TREATMENT

A few general words before describing the specifics of treatment. Therapy for syphilis differs from that for gonorrhea in two important ways. First, it is the stage and not the location of disease that governs treatment; a primary chancre in the mouth or rectum gets equal treatment. Secondly, there is no problem of penicillin resistance. The only situations in which a patient should not be given penicillin are if he is allergic to it or is being treated for another infection with an antibiotic that will simultaneously cure syphilis.

Treatment can fail if inadequate doses are given, either because the stage was misjudged or because the patient didn't take the full course of antibiotics. Reinfection is, however, much more common than treatment failure.

The main drug used for almost all stages of syphilis is benzathine penicillin, which is given as an intramuscular injection. It is much longer-acting than procaine penicillin, the form used to treat gonorrhea, and the two are not interchangeable. Only if the patient has incubating syphilis and his VDRL is still negative will the treatment of gonorrhea with penicillin be killing two birds with one stone; after that, syphilis has to be specifically treated.

Patients who have syphilis can get an unusual reaction within hours of taking penicillin. Fifty percent of those who have primary syphilis and 90 percent of those with secondary get a flu-like syndrome that includes fever, headache, and muscle aches and pains starting a few hours after taking penicillin and subsiding within 12 to 24 hours. Called a Jarisch-Herxheimer reaction, it results from a sudden breakup of the bacteria and not from an adverse reaction to the antibiotic. Aspirin and bed rest usually control the symptoms; very rarely, a more severe reaction requires medical attention.

After treatment, particularly for those patients not treated with penicillin, follow-up VDRLs are very important.

The following are specific treatment recommendations from the Centers for Disease Control issued in 1982. The New York City Board of Health has somewhat different recommendations; any questions should be addressed to the treating physician.

Early Syphilis

- Incubating, primary, secondary, and latent syphilis of less than one year's duration: Benzathine penicillin G, 2.4 million units divided into 2 intramuscular injections, both given during a single visit.

  For penicillin-allergic patients: Tetracycline HCL, 500mg four times a day for fifteen days. For those unable to tolerate tetracycline: Erythromycin, 500mg four times a day for fifteen days.

Late Syphilis

- Syphilis of more than one year's duration (except neurosyphilis) or latent syphilis of indeterminate duration: Benzathine penicillin G, 2.4 million units once a week for three consecutive weeks.
  Penicillin-allergic patients: Tetracycline HCL, 500mg four times a day for thirty days. If unable to tolerate tetracycline, then erythromycin, 500mg four times a day for thirty days.
- Neurosyphilis: It is now thought that aqueous penicillin is better than benzathine penicillin. Aqueous crystalline penicillin G, 12 to 24 million units per day intravenously for ten days; then benzathine penicillin, 2.4 million units intramuscularly once a week for three weeks; or

  Aqueous procaine penicillin, 2.4 million units intramuscularly daily, plus probenecid, 500mg four times a day both for ten days; then benzathine penicillin, 2.4 million units once a week for three weeks, or

  Benzathine penicillin, 2.4 million units intramuscularly, once a week for three weeks.

AFTER TREATMENT

Patients who were treated for primary syphilis and those who had a positive VDRL with incubating syphilis should have a VDRL repeated 3, 6, and 12 months after being treated. Patients who were treated for secondary syphilis should have a test after 24 months in addition to those recommended for the follow-up of primary syphilis. Anyone who was treated for another stage should discuss the issue with his doctor.

PREVENTION

The only way to avoid syphilis is to avoid sexual contact with someone who has infectious lesions. For people who have multiple sexual partners, frequent screening provides an alternative approach. There are no set rules, but someone who is moderately active may choose to have a blood test every three months. The screening interval that is appropriate, given an individual's sex life, should be discussed with his physician. If a person has syphilis, it is important that he name his recent sexual contacts so they can be treated.

Gonorrhea

Gonorrhea got its name in ancient times. The Greek physician Galen supposedly coined the word in the second century A.D. by combining the Greek words for "semen" and "flow." Albert Neisser discovered the causative bacterium in 1879; a combination of the names of the discoverer and the discovered forms the bacterium's medical name: *Neisseria gonorrhoeae.* Colloquially, the disease is often called the "clap," the "drip," or "GC"—a term derived from "gonococcus," which is another word for the bacterium that causes gonorrhea.

Unlike syphilis, the incidence of gonorrhea increased steadily from the 1950s through the late 1970s. Although there has been a modest decline in the number of cases reported to the Centers for Disease Control during the past few years, gonorrhea remains by far the most commonly reported infectious disease according to CDC tallies. There are roughly 1 million cases a year according to official CDC statistics, but unofficial estimates are two to three times this figure. The large discrepancy is probably due to underreporting by private physicians, although private and public health officials alike are technically obligated to report the disease. But whichever figure is used, it is clear that gonorrhea remains a major health problem.

An important feature of the history of gonorrhea in the postantibiotic era is the continual emergence of resistant strains. In 1937 the *Journal of the American Medical Association* reported the first cures of gonorrhea from the use of sulfonamide antibiotics. But during World War II, doctors noted that larger and larger doses were needed to produce the same effects. The discovery of a new antibiotic, penicillin, temporarily solved the problem. But, once again, larger and larger doses became necessary to treat the infection; the dose of penicillin now prescribed is nearly 25 times the recommendation of a 1953 medical textbook. Then, in 1976, the first case of gonorrhea in the United States that was resistant to penicillin was reported. Five years later, in 1981, a case was found that could no longer be cured by the antibiotic used to treat penicillin-resistant strains. So far, however, all cases have been curable with some available antibiotic.

While penicillin-resistant gonorrhea is relatively uncommon among gay men compared to straight men, the situation could change. The story of gonorrhea in the Far East illustrates just how fast changes can occur: In 1973 in the Far East, the incidence of penicillin-resistant gonorrhea was 1 percent; by 1980 it was between 35 and 50 percent. In general, the penicillin-resistant variety is still uncommon in most parts of the United States, with an overall incidence of 0.2 percent. But some areas, notably Los Angeles and Miami, have much higher rates. Because antibiotic resistance develops at such fast rates and with marked regional variability, public-health experts have to keep close tabs on local changes. Wherever the penicillin-resistant variety accounts for more than 25 to 30 percent of infections, as it now does in Korea, Thailand, and Singapore, penicillin is no longer the first drug of choice.

New strains can evolve quickly because the gonococcus has a rapid reproductive rate. The process of natural selection then favors those strains that are resistant to current antibiotics (because they survive despite treatment) and those strains that cause symptom-free infections (because they are less likely to prompt antibiotic therapy). Since people with symptomless gonorrhea are less likely to receive treatment but are equally contagious, they are very likely to spread the infection to their sexual contacts. Particularly in an era when many people have multiple sexual partners, the emergence of new strains that don't cause symptoms fosters widespread infection.

While penicillin resistance is less of a problem for gay men than it is for the general population, a bacterium that is closely related to the gonococcus seems to be more prevalent in the gay community than it is among heterosexuals. *Neisseria meningitidis,* also called meningococcus, was found in 35 to 42 percent of gay men, as opposed to 6 to 15 percent of straight men. The significance of this finding is not entirely clear. In the mouth the meningococcus doesn't

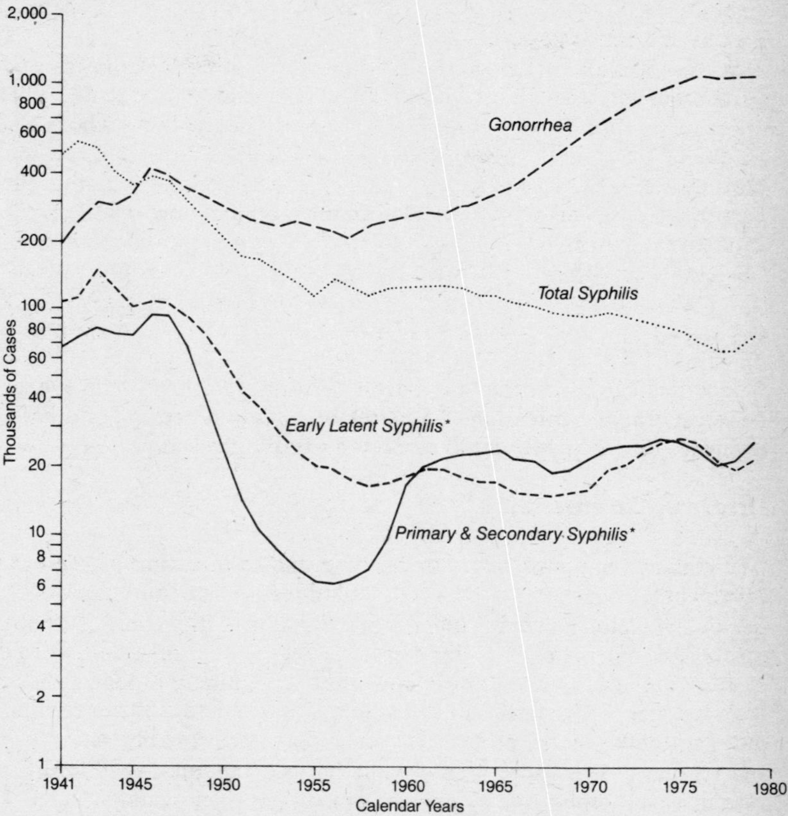

*1941-1946 Fiscal Years: Twelve month period ending June 30 of years speciified. 1947-1979 Calendar Years.

Source: CDC 9.688, HHS:PHS:CDC:CPS:VDCD: Atlanta, Georgia 30333

Syphilis and gonorrhea, reported cases by diagnosis in United States for calendar years 1941–1979

cause symptoms and doesn't need treatment; in the urethra and rectum, it can occasionally cause symptoms that require antibiotics. Luckily, the drugs that cure gonococcal urethritis will also cure meningococcal urethritis and proctitis.

When talking about gonorrhea—its symptoms, diagnosis, and cure—one has to specify what part of the body is infected. This approach differs from the one used to describe syphilis, where the length of time that one has had the infection is usually more important than what anatomical part is infected. In discussing the treatment of gonorrhea, it is also important to know whether the causative strain is resistant to penicillin; this, too, is different from the situation with syphilis, where penicillin resistance is unheard of.

SYMPTOMS

Gonorrhea can infect the urethra, the rectum, the throat, the eye, or be a generalized infection. The sites of infection are not mutually exclusive; one or more can be infected at any given time.

Urethral Gonorrhea

The classic symptoms of gonorrhea are due to infection of the urethra, the tube that connects the bladder to the outside world. Patients develop burning and frequency of urination, and a penile discharge that varies from cream-colored to yellow or green. While studies of heterosexual men show that a significant portion may have no symptoms from urethral gonorrhea, 90 to 100 percent of gay men do have symptoms. This difference is probably related to the strains of the bacteria prevalent in each community. The high rate of very bothersome symptoms among gay men usually leads to prompt treatment, which has made complications of urethral gonorrhea rare.

When complications occur, they are due to the scarring left by inflammation, or to the spread of the infection to other parts of the genital tract that connect with the urethra. Urethral scarring causes a "stricture"—a narrowing of the tube. This blocks the flow of urine and results in a diminished stream and urinary discomfort. If infection spreads to parts of the genital tract that are conduits for sperm, scarring can also cause sterility. Gonococcal urethritis can also cause epididymitis, which results in testicular pain and swelling. But

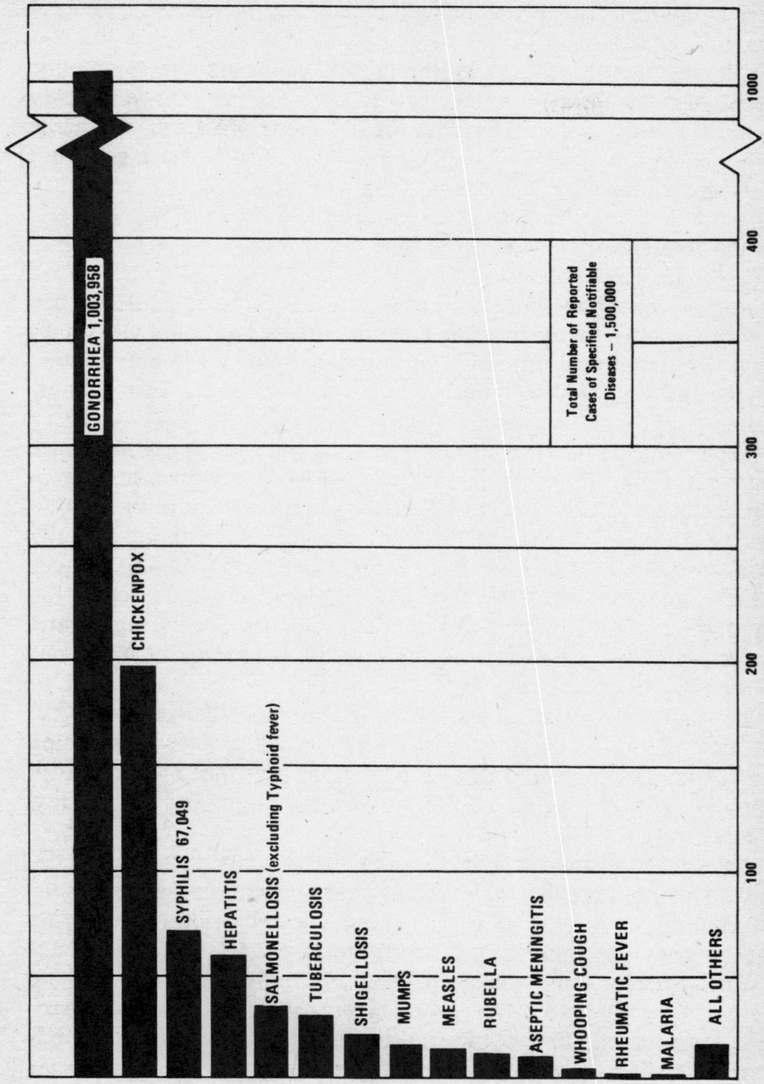

Communicable diseases—number of reported cases in United States for calendar year 1979

Source: U.S. Department of Health and Human Services, Public Health Service, Centers for Disease Control

these complications do not arise if gonorrhea is treated promptly with antibiotics.

Although nongonococcal urethritis can cause similar symptoms, the discharge is usually thinner and its color lighter. However, only laboratory tests can reliably distinguish nongonococcal urethritis from gonococcal urethritis—simply looking at the discharge is not an adequate way of making a diagnosis.

Anorectal Gonorrhea

Anorectal gonorrhea poses a more considerable problem for gay men because as many as two-thirds of infections cause no symptoms. Since patients without symptoms usually don't get treated, they act as a reservoir of unsuspected disease that is easily transmitted.

When rectal gonorrhea does cause symptoms, patients may have severe complaints or rather minor discomfort. Some men develop an anal discharge, blood and pus in the stool, burning pain in the rectum, pain on defecation, and an urge to defecate without actually having to do so. Others develop anal and perianal itching, mucus in the stool, and slight staining of underwear. In either case, the symptoms may abate without antibiotics, leaving an asymptomatic carrier—someone who has no symptoms but who remains infectious for others.

The symptoms of rectal gonorrhea are not specific for this infection but may be caused by a wide variety of problems including amebiasis, herpes, syphilis, granuloma inguinale, chancroid, lymphogranuloma venereum, *Chlamydia* infection, and mechanical trauma—only laboratory tests will tell.

The sort of complications seen with rectal gonorrhea usually depend on whether the original infection did or didn't cause symptoms. Symptomatic rectal infection can cause a rectal stricture—scarring that narrows the rectum and therefore obstructs defecation. But most people with symptoms get treated promptly and rarely develop this problem. Symptom-free rectal gonorrhea, on the other hand, may go untreated. This allows the bacteria to spread to the bloodstream, causing a generalized infection and creating problems at distant sites. The problems of a generalized infection will shortly be described.

Oral Gonorrhea

Although there is no question that the gonococcus can infect the throat, there is little agreement on the significance of this fact. Roughly 90 percent of patients with gonococcal throat infections have no symptoms, although occasionally they develop sore throats or tonsillitis. The question is whether an unsuspected case can lead to a generalized infection for the patient or can cause urethral or rectal infection in a sexual partner through fellatio or anilingus. While symptom-free rectal gonorrhea can cause a generalized infection and can also cause problems for partners, oral gonorrhea has been suspected of doing both but has not been proven to do either.

Gonorrhea of the Eye

Conjunctivitis is an inflammation of the outer layer of the eye, causing "pink-eye" and puslike discharge. The symptoms are basically the same regardless of the cause of inflammation. Gonococcal conjunctivitis acquired by infants passing through the birth canal and called "ophthalmia neonatorum" was the reason for giving silver nitrate eye drops to newborns. But adults with gonorrhea can also spread the infection to their eyes. Because this can lead to destruction of the cornea, it needs to be diagnosed and treated promptly.

Generalized Gonorrhea

Most people who get gonorrhea get only local symptoms at the site of inoculation with the bacteria: For example, a man with rectal gonorrhea who practices anal-receptive intercourse will give his insertive partner urethral gonorrhea. But 2 to 3 percent of patients with gonorrhea get generalized or "disseminated" infections because the gonococci enter the bloodstream and are transported to distant sites within the body. A generalized infection is most likely to occur in someone whose initial infection caused no symptoms, or caused symptoms that were too minor to prompt medical attention. Classically, this occurred in women with cervical infections because cervical gonorrhea is often symptomless. But as asymptomatic rectal gonorrhea among gay men has become a growing problem, men now account for a rising proportion of disseminated gonococcal infections. In 1977 in New York City, there were three times as many cases in women as in men; by 1979 the ratio dropped to 1.5:1. This shift reflects both the introduction of screening programs for women and the rising number of asymptomatic infections in men.

There is evidence that differences in bacterial strains and in individual immunological susceptibility (particularly in patients who get recurrent infections) also play a role in determining whether a local infection will become generalized. Disseminated gonorrhea tends to be caused by more-virulent strains of the bacteria. But, luckily, these strains are usually very sensitive to penicillin, and hence easily cured.

Disseminated gonorrhea often begins with nonspecific symptoms: shaking chills and fever—the result of bacteria circulating in the blood. The most common specific symptoms are a skin rash and arthritis; because the two often go together, they are known as the "arthritis-dermatitis syndrome."

The rash consists of tiny spots, sometimes filled with pus, usually found near the hands and feet and asymmetrically distributed over the right and left halves of the body (unlike the rash of syphilis, which is symmetrical). The rash usually heals within a matter of days.

The arthritis typically affects the ankles, wrists, knees, elbows, and small joints of the hands and feet. Usually several joints ache before one becomes red and swollen. While the diagnosis of gonococcal arthritis tends to be straightforward, other illnesses can mimic the symptoms, particularly one called "Reiter's syndrome," which also causes a urethritis, arthritis, and conjunctivitis. The cause of Reiter's syndrome is unknown, and gonorrhea should always be excluded by proper laboratory testing.

Since the advent of antibiotics, the two most serious complications of disseminated gonorrhea—heart disease and meningitis—have become very rare. The heart disease—with infection of the heart valves (endocarditis), inflammation of the heart muscle (myocarditis) and lining around the heart (pericarditis)—and meningitis are usually preceded by the joint and skin symptoms, which if treated promptly do not progress to the more serious complications.

TRANSMISSION

Sexual contact with an infected partner is the usual mode of transmission; it is estimated that the chances are between 50 and 80 percent of catching gonorrhea from one act of intercourse with an infected partner. Infants can catch it on their way out of the birth canal, but sexual abuse should be suspected if a child has gonorrhea. Only human beings harbor this bacterium, which requires warmth and moisture to survive and therefore cannot live outside the body for long. While toilet-seat transmission is theoretically possible if a man's penis touches a discharge recently left on the seat by someone else, this is a very unlikely way to catch it.

The incubation period—that stretch of time between contact and developing symptoms—is two to ten days. But unlike syphilis, there is no "safe period" between catching the infection and being able to pass it on. Within hours of sexual contact, a previously uninfected person can transmit the infection to a new partner.

DIAGNOSIS

The two laboratory tests used to diagnose gonorrhea are the Gram stain and culture. Whether one or both of these tests should be done depends on which anatomical site is being screened. Each location needs to be evaluated separately, although as a rule most people who are tested for gonorrhea get oral, urethral, and rectal tests. The Gram stain involves putting a sample of the urethral or rectal discharge on a slide, staining it with certain dyes, and then looking at it under the microscope. A positive test is one where "Gram-negative intracellular diplococci" are seen—this is the medical description of the pink-colored, kidney-shaped bacteria that can be seen inside pus cells. The results of the Gram stain are ready in minutes.

A culture requires putting a sample on a growth medium and then incubating it for a couple of days. It is more specific than a Gram stain (only the culture will differentiate between gonococcus and meningococcus), but the results take longer. A special culture medium, the Thayer-Martin one, is used to grow the gonococcus, but some reports suggest that changes in bacterial strains over the past two years may necessitate changes in this standard procedure. It is now recommended that positive cultures be tested for the enzyme B-lactamase that makes gonorrhea resistant to penicillin.

Urethral Gonorrhea

The Gram stain, if positive, is sufficient to make this diagnosis. The test can be done on the urethral discharge or on a centrifuged specimen of urine. Cultures are necessary only if the Gram stain is negative, if this is a repeat bout of urethritis after the patient has recently been treated, or if the penicillin-resistant strains are prevalent in this part of the country. But rectal and throat cultures will probably also be done because patients may have simultaneous infections at these sites. Since most gay men with gonococcal urethritis have symptoms, taking urethral cultures from men with neither symptoms nor a history of contact is not generally necessary.

Anorectal Gonorrhea

Both the Gram stain and the culture are useful in a patient with symptoms. Using an anoscope—a roughly three-inch instrument inserted into the rectum—the mucous membrane lining the rectum is looked at and samples of the discharge removed with cotton swabs for the two tests. If the Gram stain is positive or the patient has had a known contact, he should be treated immediately; otherwise he should wait for the culture report.

The Gram stain is less useful for diagnosing symptomless patients, in whom a culture, taken simply by inserting a cotton swab—without the anoscope—should be done. Routine rectal screening of sexually active men who are not in exclusive, monogamous relationships, and who have rectal intercourse or engage in anilingus, is worthwhile because a significant number have symptom-free infections that can be transmitted, causing disease in sexual partners.

Oral Gonorrhea

Gram stains for GC of the throat are useless because some of the bacteria that normally live in the throat have an appearance similar to GC. Diagnosis can only be made by throat culture. Men who have infections at other sites and those who have had contact with infected partners should be tested. But some investigators feel that routine screening for gonorrhea should not include a throat culture in men who are being tested simply because they are sexually active rather than because they have symptoms or because they know that they have had contact with someone who has gonorrhea.

Gonorrhea of the Eye

The discharge should be Gram-stained and cultured.

Generalized Gonorrhea

Any discharge should be Gram-stained and all possible sites should be cultured. Additional tests include blood cultures and taking fluid from swollen joints or pus from the rash for Gram stain and culture. Even if the blood cultures and joint fluids are negative for GC—as they are in 50 percent of cases—disseminated gonorrhea is the presumptive diagnosis in anyone with localized gonorrhea who then develops arthritis. Treatment should be started, and improvement of symptoms within 48 hours helps confirm the diagnosis.

TREATMENT

Choosing the correct antibiotic depends on where the infection is located and whether another STD is going to be treated at the same time. A few general words about certain antibiotics that are often used to treat gonorrhea: Procaine penicillin can cure incubating syphilis; tetracycline will cure chlamydial infections that frequently accompany gonorrhea, but it is not recommended for rectal gonorrhea; ampicillin and amoxicillin are not recommended for rectal or oral gonorrhea; and spectinomycin won't cure oral gonorrhea.

The following are the latest 1982 Centers for Disease Control recommendations. But there are other treatments available and, remember, antibiotic sensitivities change.

Urethral Gonorrhea

Penicillin. Probenecid, 1 gram by mouth to raise blood levels of penicillin. Then, aqueous procaine penicillin G, 4.8 million units divided into two intramuscular injections given during one visit.

Advantages: single treatment; cures incubating syphilis, oral and rectal gonorrhea.

Disadvantages: doesn't cure chlamydial infections, which are another common cause of urethritis and which may coexist with the gonococcal infection.

Other antibiotics:

Tetracycline HCl, 500mg orally, four times a day for seven days. (Tetracycline should not be taken with milk products or with antacids since these interfere with absorption of the drug.)

Advantages: for patients who are allergic to procaine or penicillin.

An allergic reaction to penicillin has different symptoms from an adverse reaction to procaine. The first consists of hives, itching, or wheezing, whereas the second consists of agitation, disorientation, or hallucinations. Tetracycline also cures chlamydial infections (although this dose may not be sufficient for chlamydial infections) and oral gonorrhea.

Disadvantages: it may not cure rectal infections, and it requires taking a prolonged course of antibiotics.

Amoxicillin, 3.0 grams orally, or ampicillin, 3.5 grams orally, each with 1 gram of probenecid.

Advantages: single dose.

Disadvantages: doesn't cure chlamydia, anorectal or oral gonorrhea.

Anorectal Gonorrhea

Aqueous procaine penicillin G, same dose as for urethral, or:

Spectinomycin, 2.0 grams in one intramuscular injection. Advantages: cures penicillin-resistant GC. Disadvantages: does not cure throat infections.

A word about using tetracycline for anorectal gonorrhea: It should not be used unless test-of-cure cultures are taken after treatment because it fails to cure 15 to 20 percent of anorectal gonococcal infections.

Oral Gonorrhea

Penicillin or tetracycline, in the same doses used for urethral GC.

Gonorrhea of the Eye

Patients should be hospitalized, treated with aqueous crystalline penicillin G, 10 million units intravenously daily for five days. Eyes should be rinsed with normal saline hourly until the discharge disappears.

Generalized Gonorrhea

Usually patients are hospitalized; those with endocarditis or meningitis need additional treatment.

Aqueous crystalline penicillin G, 10 million units daily, until symptoms improve, then amoxicillin or ampicillin, 500 mg orally, four times a day to complete at least one week of antibiotic treatment.

Oral regimens include the use of amoxicillin, ampicillin, tetracycline, or erythromycin for at least seven days.

AFTER TREATMENT

Infected sites should be recultured four to seven days after finishing treatment. These are known as "test-of-cure" cultures; they are designed to see whether the treatment was successful. There are several reasons why treatment may fail. The first is that the patient didn't finish the full course of antibiotics; the second is that he was treated with penicillin for a penicillin-resistant infection. But the third reason that test-of-cure cultures may be positive is the most common reason: The patient got reinfected. Technically, this isn't a failure of treatment but a new infection that requires another course of antibiotics.

If treatment fails, the bacteria should be tested for penicillin resistance and the patient treated with spectinomycin. If this fails, the bacteria should be tested for spectinomycin resistance and the patient treated with cefoxitin, 2.0 grams intramuscularly, and probenecid, 1 gram orally, or cefotaxime, 1 gram intramuscularly, and probenecid. Since neither spectinomycin nor cefoxitin works against oral gonorrhea, treatment with another antibiotic, trimethoprim/sulfamethoxazole, is needed for throat infections due to penicillin-resistant gonorrhea.

PREVENTION

The only way to avoid gonorrhea is to avoid sexual contact with someone who has the infection. But several strategies will help control this infection in the community and also offer personal benefits. Someone who has multiple partners, particularly in an anonymous setting, should be screened periodically for gonorrhea—particularly for asymptomatic rectal infections if his sexual practices involve rectal contact. The intervals at which this should be done are variable and should be discussed with the doctor. Anyone who has gonorrhea should name his contacts during the past two weeks so that they can be treated immediately. And anyone who knows that he has had contact with someone who has gonorrhea should be tested and treated for the infection.

Urinating after sex may decrease the likelihood of catching urethral gonorrhea, but the benefits have not been scientifically proven.

Finally, a vaccine against gonorrhea is being studied.

THE MINOR STDS

Viral Diseases: Warts and Molluscum Contagiosum
Tropical Diseases: Lymphogranuloma Venereum, Granuloma Inguinale, and Chancroid
Infestations: Pubic Lice and Scabies

Minor STDs can be major aggravations. That these diseases are called "minor" is a medical judgment about their consequences, which are usually restricted to the genital or rectal areas, unlike such diseases as syphilis, which can inflict its ravages on many of the body's organs. Several of the minor STDs are also "minor" in the sense that they afflict relatively few persons in the United States.

Minor STDs fall into three basic classes: those caused by viruses (genital warts and molluscum contagiosum); those that are traditionally "tropical" diseases (lymphogranuloma venereum, granuloma inguinale, and chancroid); and those that are actually infestations rather than infections (scabies and crabs).

Because minor STDs cause symptoms that usually prompt a doctor's visit and because they are frequently found in patients who have other STDs, many health authorities suggest that this is an excellent opportunity to screen for syphilis and gonorrhea.

THE VIRAL DISEASES: WARTS AND MOLLUSCUM CONTAGIOSUM

Venereal Warts

Many people who have had genital or rectal warts can attest to the fact that they can be a major inconvenience. It isn't that they cause severe symptoms but rather that the need for prolonged treatment can be a costly and time-consuming ritual of frequent visits to the doctor.

All warts are skin tumors caused by the *Papillomavirus*. Different warts have different medical names, depending on their shape and location. Venereal warts are called "condylomata acuminata." They are flesh-colored, there are usually several at one time, and they can coalesce to form large, cauliflower-like lesions. They have a marked predilection for warm, moist areas—hence their location.

Although the virus that causes anogenital warts looks the same as the virus that causes common skin warts when it is examined under an electron microscope, the concentration of the virus in anogenital warts is very low compared with that of warts in other areas.

While it isn't really known how common warts are, a survey by the Centers for Disease Control that sampled random visits to STD clinics showed that there were 33 cases for each 1000 patient visits.

Warts are located on the penile shaft, under the foreskin, in the anus, and in the perianal region. They can also occur in the urethral opening and in the mouth. Uncircumcised men have more penile warts than circumcised men. But among gay men, anal warts are five to ten times more common than genital warts.

Genital warts rarely cause symptoms (other than being visible), but anal warts can cause itching and bleeding with anal intercourse or after bowel movements. A rare complication of very large warts is that they can become malignant.

Venereal warts are sexually transmitted. The usual incubation period is two to three months, but symptoms can develop from one month to one year after exposure. Approximately 60 percent of persons exposed to venereal warts develop them. However, despite repeated exposure, some people never do. This variation in susceptibility is probably due to differences in natural immunity.

While anal warts are also presumed to be sexually transmitted and are said to correlate with anal-receptive intercourse, no one really understands their transmission. The problem is that few of the insertive partners seem to have penile warts, making it difficult to understand how the receptive partner got his anal warts.

The diagnosis of warts is usually a clinical one: it's a wart because it looks like a wart. If there is any question about the diagnosis because the lesion looks unusual, a biopsy should be done. The wart is removed and sent to a pathologist, who examines it under the microscope.

While genital warts are obvious, anal warts may be hidden unless an anoscopic examination is done. A small instrument, the anoscope, is inserted into the rectum, allowing the doctor to look for (and then treat) the anal warts. Anyone with warts near the rectum should have an internal exam because of the high likelihood that internal warts will also be present. All sexual partners of patients with venereal warts should be examined for the presence of warts.

Before discussing the specifics of treatment, two general points should be emphasized. Repeated treatments are the rule rather than the exception, requiring weekly or biweekly visits until the warts disappear. Although warts sometimes go away by themselves, they can't be counted on to do so. The second point is that the sooner they are treated, the better the outcome will be. Warts only become harder to cure as they grow larger and more numerous.

Several forms of treatment are available. Podophyllin is the most widely used form of treatment, possibly because the doctor needs no special equipment—just the bottle of medicine and an applicator. Podophyllin is available as a 10- to 25-percent solution that is mixed with a benzoin base, which gives the medicine its dark brown color. Podophyllin should be applied only to the warts and care should be taken to avoid the surrounding normal tissue. The first time it is used, it should be washed off after one to two hours; subsequently, it should be left on for four to six hours and then washed off. If it is used to treat internal warts, no washing is needed. Only 50 percent of patients are cured by the first or second treatment; the rest need re-treatment every one to two weeks until the warts are gone.

Podophyllin should not be used on very large or bleeding warts, because this can lead to absorption of significant amounts into the bloodstream. High blood levels of podophyllin cause serious neurological damage, including confusion, coma, and even death.

Small warts can also be removed by freezing them with liquid nitrogen, a procedure known as "cryocautery," or by applying an acid such as trichloracetic acid.

Large warts don't respond as well to these forms of therapy. Burning them off, a technique known as "electrodesiccation," or scraping them off, a procedure called "curettage," gives better results. Both procedures are done under local anesthesia and both can cause several weeks of postoperative discomfort.

Giant warts need to be removed surgically under general anesthesia.

Molluscum Contagiosum

Molluscum contagiosum (MC) is similar to warts: it is a viral skin disease that causes small growths. MC is caused by a different virus, a poxvirus—a member of the family of viruses that includes smallpox. Unlike warts, which prefer the actual genitals or rectum, MC has a predilection for the surrounding skin rather than the mucous membranes of the genitalia or rectum.

The growths of MC are skin-colored or pearly white. They occur singly or in clusters and range in size from one millimeter to one centimeter. The salient feature of these lesions is that they have a spot in the center—like a bugbite or blackhead—through which a milky white substance can be squeezed. Unless the lesions become secondarily infected with bacteria, MC causes no symptoms. Even if untreated, many, if not most, of the growths disappear within six to nine months. Some cases, however, have been reported to persist for years.

The incubation period of this disease is two weeks to two months. MC is transmitted from person to person through direct body contact, but the patient can then spread the virus from one part of his body to another.

As with warts, the diagnosis is usually a clinical one: It's MC because that's what it looks like. If the diagnosis is in doubt, the lesions can be biopsied or the milky substance can be squeezed from the center, stained with a Giemsa stain, and examined under the microscope.

Unlike warts, MC is an easy disease to treat. Several methods of treatment are available. Two that are commonly used are scraping off the lesions (curettage) and freezing them with liquid nitrogen (cryocautery).

Patients should return to the doctor one month after treatment to make sure that there are no new growths. Sexual partners should be examined and treated if necessary.

THE TROPICAL DISEASES: LYMPHOGRANULOMA VENEREUM, GRANULOMA INGUINALE, AND CHANCROID

As the title suggests, these diseases are much more common in the tropics. Because they are fairly rare in the United States, many doctors may be unfamiliar with them and therefore have some difficulty in recognizing them.

Lymphogranuloma Venereum (LGV)

Only 199 cases of LGV were reported to the Centers for Disease Control in 1980. This rare disease is caused by a small bacterium known as *Chlamydia trachomatis,* a bacterium that is better known for causing nongonococcal urethritis and trachoma eye infections. Of *Chlamydia*'s 15 strains, only three—L-1, L-2, and L-3—cause LGV. But these three strains invade tissues more readily than the ones that cause other chlamydial diseases.

The first sign of LGV is a painless, innocuous lesion on the genitals or in the rectum. It is usually dismissed as a pimple; in fact, 50 percent of patients cannot recall having had the lesions even after they are diagnosed as having the disease.

Two to three weeks later, the hallmark of LGV appears: painful, swollen lymph nodes in the groin caused by spread of the infection through the lymph channels. These nodes, called "buboes," occur on only one side in two-thirds of patients. The other one-third develop the swelling on both sides of the groin. At first the lymph nodes are movable; but as the disease spreads, the overlying skin becomes red and sticks to the nodes. As the nodes enlarge, a classic sign of LGV develops—the "sign of the groove." The groove is created by a ligament that runs across the lymph nodes in the groin, which fails to stretch as the nodes grow larger on either side. Eventually, the lymph nodes soften and discharge their fluid, which contains blood and pus, through the overlying skin. During this phase of LGV, most people have general signs of illness: fever, headache, and joint pains. While the nonspecific symptoms subside without treatment, the buboes don't.

If LGV affects the rectum, as it can in anyone practicing anal intercourse, widespread inflammation can occur with all the symptoms of proctitis—the urge to defecate and a rectal discharge containing blood and pus. Because other, much more common infections, such as gonorrhea, cause proctitis, they should be excluded before the diagnosis of LGV is made. This follows a familiar medical adage: "If you hear hoofbeats, think of horses, not zebras."

Untreated LGV can cause severe long-term complications because the severe inflammation produces scarring. The complications are rectal strictures, which block bowel movements; perirectal abscesses; fistulas, which are abnormal canals between one internal organ and another or between an internal organ and the skin; and severe genital swelling because of blocked lymph channels.

LGV is known to be a sexually transmitted disease with a fairly short incubation period; the pimple usually develops seven to twelve days after exposure.

The diagnosis is usually suspected during the swollen-node stage. The laboratory test most widely used to confirm the diagnosis is a blood test that measures the level of complement-fixing antibodies. An antibody level greater than 1:32, and usually greater than 1:64, is the standard of diagnosis. Unfortunately, the test is somewhat nonspecific because it includes antibodies against all strains of *Chlamydia,* including the ones that cause urethritis and eye infections. However, antibody levels tend not to rise as high with other chlamydial infections as they do with LGV.

A more specific antibody test, the microimmunofluorescent test, is available, but there are also problems with its use. The only way to actually prove the diagnosis is by culturing fluid withdrawn from a softened lymph node; however, cultures for *Chlamydia* are still not routine at many laboratories. In practical terms, most doctors decide to treat LGV on the basis of symptoms and the complement-fixing-antibody test.

The sooner LGV is treated, the better the outcome. Antibiotics will decrease the inflammation, but they can't undo scarring.

Tetracycline, 500mg orally, four times a day for two to three weeks is the treatment of choice. Often two or more courses of therapy are needed. The success of treatment is gauged by the appearance of the lymph nodes, which should shrink and not hurt.

Large, soft lymph nodes should also be drained by withdrawing the fluid through a needle. They should not be cut open, since this only increases scarring.

Because the disease can recur, patients should be examined and have their LGV antibody levels checked every three months for one year after treatment ends.

Granuloma Inguinale

In many ways granuloma inguinale is similar to LGV. It is common in the tropics, particularly in the Caribbean, New Guinea, and Southeast Asia. It causes an initial sore that is inconspicuous, but if untreated, causes extensive tissue destruction. The infection is rare in the United States; only 51 cases were reported to the Centers for Disease Control in 1980.

Granuloma inguinale is caused by a bacterium that looks like a closed safety pin and was discovered by Charles Donovan in 1905. The disease is sometimes still called donovanosis, but the bacterium, which was originally named after its discoverer, has been renamed *Calymmatobacterium granulomatis.*

The first symptom of granuloma inguinale is a bump that is usually located on the genitals, thigh, or near the rectum, but can occur in the mouth or elsewhere on the skin. The lesion bleeds easily and may itch, but it isn't painful. Frequently it causes no discomfort and patients wait months before seeking medical care. The bump then develops into an ulcer that smells bad, has a beefy-red color, and steadily enlarges. This is the chronic stage of the disease.

Untreated granuloma inguinale can destroy local tissues, causing deformity of the genitals or rectum. Prompt treatment with antibiotics prevents this, but it does not reverse damage caused by scarring.

The evidence that granuloma inguinale is sexually transmitted is circumstantial. The disease is commonest in the most sexually active age group; there is a high rate of concomitant syphilis; and the lesions are usually located on the genitals of straight men and often found in the rectum among gay men. The incubation period isn't accurately known but is estimated to be three to six weeks.

Diagnosing granuloma inguinale may be difficult because it is so rare in this country that most doctors have never seen it. This problem is expressed in the medical adage that "to diagnose a disease, you have to think of it first."

To test for granuloma inguinale, the lesion is scraped or biopsied and the sample then examined under the microscope, looking for white blood cells that contain the bacteria. The cells are called "Donovan bodies." A few attempts at diagnosis may be needed before these cells are spotted.

Many antibiotics can cure granuloma inguinale. Tetracycline is the one most often used. The dose is 500mg four times a day for three weeks, or longer if the lesions are not completely healed by then. Since relapses can occur, the patient should be periodically checked by his doctor for several months following the completion of therapy. Steady sex partners should also be examined and treated.

Chancroid

Chancroid is much more common in the United States than either LGV or granuloma inguinale. Nearly 800 cases are reported annually, but authorities estimate that the true number of cases is actually much higher because many cases are either misdiagnosed or not reported to the Centers for Disease Control.

The hallmark of chancroid, which is also known as the "soft chancre," is one or more extremely painful genital or anal ulcers that usually develop one to five days after exposure. The pain of chancroid helps distinguish these ulcers from those of primary syphilis, which are usually painless. But lest the two diseases be thought to be mutually exclusive, 15 percent of patients with chancroid also have syphilis.

The ulcer of chancroid has a ragged border with a grayish center that bleeds easily when scraped. One to three weeks after the start of ulcers, one-third to one-half of patients develop painful swelling of the lymph nodes in the groin. Unlike patients with LGV or primary herpes (who also have anogenital lesions and swollen nodes), patients with chancroid rarely develop general signs of infection such as fever, chills, or headache. Like the lymph nodes of LGV, those of chancroid can also become soft and fluid-filled, and the fluid can drain through to the surface.

Chancroid is caused by the bacterium *Haemophilus ducreyi*. But the organism is a tricky one to find. An effort should be made by taking a sample of the ulcer or by withdrawing fluid from a soft lymph node and looking under the microscope for small, Gram-negative rods with rounded ends that are arranged in bands of parallel rows, an arrangement that has been likened to a "school of fish." But even if the test is accurately done, it only detects 50 percent of cases, and cultures for the bacteria remain impractical.

Chancroid is thus often a diagnosis of exclusion. It's what's left after LGV, syphilis, herpes, and granuloma inguinale are ruled out by appropriate tests.

The treatment of chancroid now recommended by the Centers for Disease Control represents a change from that listed in standard medical textbooks. The first drug of choice is erythromycin, 500mg four times a day for at least ten days, or until the ulcers are healed. An alternative is trimethoprim/sulfamethoxazole, 160/800mg

(Septra or Bactrim DS) twice a day for the same time period. All sexual partners should be treated with one of these drugs for ten days.

If there are large lymph nodes that have become soft and contain fluid, these should be drained using a needle that is inserted into the nodes, being careful to puncture only normal skin.

THE INFESTATIONS: PUBIC LICE AND SCABIES

Pubic Lice

Pubic lice are known colloquially as "crabs" and scientifically as *Phthirus pubis*. The louse has three pairs of legs that end in sharp claws; a pair of stubby antennae; and no wings. The pubic louse is closely related to head and body lice, but the latter two are varieties of a different louse known as *Pediculus humanus*. Pubic lice don't infest the scalp, because their mating habits require hairs that are relatively far apart from one another.

The main symptom of pubic lice is itching in the anogenital region. The itching is worse at night and develops as a response both to the puncture wound inflicted by the crab and to the digestive juices and fecal material that the crab injects into its host.

The infestation can spread to the thighs, armpits, beard, and eyelashes. Patients may see the crabs or the nits—the eggs, which seem glued to the hairs. While crabs are naturally light gray, they can turn brown from sucking the victim's blood, giving them the appearance of tiny scabs.

Pubic lice are almost always caught from sexual partners. They are said to be the most highly contagious STD because of the 95 percent chance of getting them from one sexual encounter with an infested mate. Since the louse can survive for 24 hours on sheets, towels, and clothes, crabs can be caught indirectly, but this is a very unusual way of acquiring them.

To diagnose crabs, the itchy area should be carefully inspected with the aid of a magnifying hand lens. If there is a problem seeing either the crabs or the nits, a hair can be plucked and examined under the microscope.

The main prescription medication used to treat crabs is gamma-benzene hexachloride (GBH), also known as lindane, and perhaps more familiar under the trade name Kwell. It is available as a shampoo, cream, or lotion. The shampoo should be applied to the affected and adjacent areas, lathered for four minutes, and then washed off. The cream or lotion should be left on for eight to twenty-four hours and then rinsed off. This may not remove the nits, which tend to adhere to the hairs; a fine-tooth comb can be used to pry them loose.

Lindane is a potentially harmful drug if it is left on the skin too long (because it can be absorbed through the skin) or if it is swallowed. Seizures have been reported after its use. It should also never be used near the eyes. If eyelashes are infested with crabs, an ophthalmic ointment should be applied to the lids twice a day for ten days. This will smother the lice.

A nonprescription drug that contains pyrethrins and piperonyl butoxide, whose trade name is Rid, was found to be as effective as Kwell in one study. Rid should be applied to the affected and adjacent areas, left on for ten minutes, and then washed off. Rid shouldn't be used by anyone with ragweed allergies.

Recent sexual partners of persons with crabs should also be treated. Clothing and bed linens that have been used within the past two days should be washed in very hot water or dry-cleaned.

Scabies

Scabies is caused by a mite, *Sarcoptes scabiei,* which belongs to the Arachnida class of insects, a group that also includes spiders and scorpions. Unlike crabs, which stay on the skin's surface, the female mite burrows her way under the skin, where she lays her eggs. While a single mite can cause a case of scabies, ten mites are the average in a typical case.

Like pubic lice, the hallmark of scabies is also itching that is worse at night. The itching develops in those places where the female digs her tracks. She has a predilection for finger webs, wrists, and the genital region, but she can also infest the feet, elbows, armpits, buttocks, and nipples. The burrows are visible as thin, raised, grayish lines that look like small splinters with an average length of ten millimeters. If the urge to scratch is readily indulged, the lesions can become infected by bacteria. Such infection is the main complication of scabies.

For the person with his first case of scabies, itching doesn't start until a month after infestation because the itching is due to an allergic reaction to the mite and her products. During the first episode, it takes time for the allergic reacton to develop; during subsequent infestations, the allergic reaction occurs much more quickly. Persons with repeat infestations usually start to itch within 24 hours.

Scabies is primarily transmitted by close personal contact. Sixty to 80 percent of cases are caught from sexual partners. However, it is the close contact and not the sexual activity that is responsible. Since the mite can survive on sheets and towels for two to three days, inanimate objects can transmit the infestation.

The diagnosis of scabies depends on finding the mite, which lies hidden in its burrow. After putting a drop of mineral oil on the burrow, the burrow is scraped with a scalpel, and a sample is then examined under the microscope. Any history of itching in the mite's preferred locations, coupled with the patient's knowing others who have a similar itch, should prompt a thorough search for scabies.

Scabies is also treated with Kwell. The cream or lotion should be applied to the entire body from the neck down, left on for 8 to 24 hours, and then washed off. Some doctors think a second application should routinely be used one week later because Kwell won't kill the mite's eggs. Since the eggs would have hatched in the intervening week, they would be susceptible to the second application. Other doctors disagree and think that one treatment should suffice.

Most people get relief within 48 hours of treatment, but there are several reasons why symptoms may persist. Kwell can cause skin irritation; the allergic reaction to the mites may persist for several weeks after the patient is cured; and the mites may not have been eradicated. If symptoms do persist, another search for the mites should be made. If they are still present, re-treatment is in order; if there is severe skin irritation from an allergy or drug reaction, the doctor may suggest treatment with a steroid cream.

Recent sexual partners and bedmates should also be treated with Kwell. Clothing and bedding used within the past two days should be washed in hot water or dry-cleaned.

THE "ITISES": URETHRITIS (NGU), PROCTITIS, EPIDIDYMITIS, AND PROSTATITIS

"Itis" is a medical suffix that means inflammation. When "itis" is appended to the name of an anatomical part, it means that the organ is inflamed. "Colitis" denotes an inflamed colon, and "urethritis" an inflamed urethra—to mention but two examples of "itises."

Stating that an organ is inflamed doesn't explain why it is inflamed. When trying to determine what has caused the inflammation, there are two principles worth remembering. First, the causes of inflammation fall into three basic categories: infection, trauma, and unknown causes (in which case the body is thought to cause inflammation because of some internal derangement). Second, each organ has its common and uncommon causes of inflammation, and it is a good idea to start by looking for the common ones first. For example, if an eye is inflamed, it is logical to look for something that flew into it; trauma would be the cause of inflammation. If the urethra were inflamed, however, it would make more sense to look for gonorrhea first, in which case infection would account for the inflammation.

Whatever produces the inflammation, the symptoms are similar: An eye irritated by a scratch may look and feel the same as one irritated by infection. It is nevertheless crucial to find out why the eye is inflamed, because only then can it be properly treated.

Urethritis (NGU)

The urethra is the channel connecting the bladder (where urine is stored) to the outside world. When it becomes inflamed, the symptoms are burning and frequency of urination, with or without a penile discharge.

The first diagnosis that should be excluded is gonorrhea. Once laboratory tests determine that gonorrhea is not the cause, the diagnosis is "nongonococcal urethritis" (NGU) or "nonspecific urethritis" (NSU). Although these terms are used interchangeably, NGU is the correct one because the urethritis may well have a specific cause that just doesn't happen to be gonorrhea.

Infection remains the most likely reason for urethritis. Most NGU is caused by two bacteria-like organisms, *Chlamydia trachomatis*—which causes 40 percent of cases—and *Ureaplasma urealyticum*—which causes 20 percent. These organisms are called "bacteria-like" because they meet some of the criteria of being a bacterium (they have a cell wall and are susceptible to antibiotics) but not all the criteria (they can't survive outside of the patient's cells).

Overall, NGU is now thought to be more common than gonococcal urethritis. Although gay men do get NGU, they seem to get it less frequently than do straight men. The suspected reason for this is that *Chlamydia* and *U. urealyticum* are less readily acquired during anal intercourse than they are from vaginal intercourse.

It is said that the symptoms of NGU are milder than those of gonococcal urethritis, that the discharge is clear or white rather than cream-colored or yellow, and that there is less discomfort when urinating. While this may be true as a general rule, it is not a reliable means of making the diagnosis. Only laboratory tests—a Gram stain and culture—can distinguish the two.

The problem of diagnosing NGU is that both *Chlamydia* and *U. urealyticum* require special cultures that are not routinely available (although they can be done in special laboratories if a patient does not get better on a standard course of antibiotics). In practical terms, NGU is diagnosed by finding urethritis without finding the gonococcus.

But patients who have gonococcal urethritis can also have NGU simultaneously. This is discovered when the symptoms of urethritis persist after the gonorrhea has been cured by penicillin. Since the incubation period of NGU is longer than that of gonorrhea, and since NGU isn't cured by penicillin, patients complain of urethritis one to two weeks after being treated for gonorrhea.

NGU is usually treated with tetracycline, although opinions differ on what the dose should be. The Centers for Disease Control recommend 500mg four times a day for at least seven days. The New York City Health Department suggests 500mg four times a day for seven days, followed by 250mg four times a day for fourteen days. The advantage of tetracycline is that it treats both urethral gonorrhea and NGU. Gay men should know, however, that tetracycline often does not cure rectal gonorrhea, and that therefore both penicillin and tetracycline may be needed.

Although infections cause most cases of urethritis, there are instances in which the cause is unknown. Reiter's syndrome, whose hallmarks are urethritis, conjunctivitis, and arthritis occurs most often in men between the ages of 20 and 40. The urethritis is the first symptom to develop, followed by conjunctivitis, which only lasts a few days, and then by arthritis, which usually affects the ankles, knees, and toes and lasts for two to four months. Most patients recover fully within one year. While sexually acquired urethritis, particularly that caused by chlamydial infection, is thought to trigger Reiter's syndrome, no one really knows what causes this disease. A particular immunologic feature seems to make certain persons susceptible to the disease, however, since 70 to 96 percent of patients have an antigen on their white blood cells known as the HLA-B 27 antigen. This antigen has been implicated in other diseases that are thought to have an immunologic basis.

Since gonorrhea can also cause urethritis, conjunctivitis, and arthritis, it is important to exclude it by laboratory testing. It may also be worthwhile to treat the urethritis with tetracycline, just in case it's caused by *Chlamydia.* But there really isn't any specific treatment for Reiter's syndrome, although antiarthritis medications may alleviate some of the discomfort caused by swollen joints.

Proctitis

Proctitis is an inflammation of the rectum. The symptoms, which vary in severity, are a rectal discharge that may contain pus and blood; rectal pain; the urge to defecate without actually having to do so; a change in bowel habits, which is often constipation but can be diarrhea; left-sided lower-abdominal pain; and, occasionally, fever.

Infections are a frequent cause of proctitis in gay men. Gonorrhea should be looked for first, by doing a Gram stain and culture. Syphilis should also be checked for by doing a blood test and, if there are ulcers in the rectum, taking a sample from them to examine under the microscope. A person found to have either gonorrhea or syphilis should be treated; if the proctitis is then cured, no further tests are necessary.

But many other infections commonly cause proctitis. Viruses can do it, particularly herpes simplex, which causes severe rectal pain. Parasitic infections also cause proctitis. While amebas, with or without *Giardia,* cause rectal inflammation, *Giardia* by itself does not cause this problem. And there is a long list of bacteria, other than syphilis and gonorrhea, that also cause proctitis: *Shigella, Salmonella, Campylobacter,* and possibly *Neisseria meningitidis.* And the bacteria-like *Chlamydia* also causes proctitis. Both the strains of *Chlamydia* that cause lymphogranuloma venereum (LGV) and the strains that cause urethritis cause chlamydial proctitis.

Trauma is another important cause of proctitis among gay men. Anal intercourse, especially without adequate lubrication; insertion of foreign objects; and fist-fornication can all irritate the rectum. Fist-fornication deserves special mention because it can rip through the full thickness of the rectal wall, requiring emergency surgery and causing serious damage—patients may need permanent colostomies. The other structural problems caused by trauma are fissures, which are small, painful tears that hurt and bleed; prolapsed hemorrhoids, which are dilated veins in the rectum that may protrude through the anus and may also hurt and bleed; and rectal abscesses, which are pockets of infection that hurt. Gay men, like anyone else, can also develop proctitis for no apparent reason. Inflammatory bowel disease, either ulcerative colitis or Crohn's disease, can cause rectal inflammation that has no known cause.

Determining which of the many possibilities is the actual reason for proctitis may take some time. The doctor should start with a careful history that includes a detailed description of symptoms; known exposure to infectious diseases; sexual practices; and whether the patient has taken any antibiotics recently, since these might affect test results and can occasionally cause bowel irritation. The physical examination should include anoscopy—a procedure in which a small instrument is inserted into the rectum, allowing the doctor to see whether there are ulcers and also to assess the severity of the inflammation. A stool smear should then be looked at under the microscope to see whether there are white blood cells, since these are not normally present and require explanation.

If the tests for syphilis and gonorrhea are negative, the order of subsequent tests depends on the physician's judgment. If infection is suspected, it is likely that *Salmonella, Shigella,* and parasites, will be tested for next, since these are common diseases. If trauma is thought to be the cause, the patient may be referred to a specialist, a proctologist. And if the cause is still not apparent after more-obscure infections are ruled out, the evaluation should proceed with sigmoidoscopy (in which a longer tube is inserted into the rectum) and possibly a rectal biopsy and X-ray studies.

While the above discussion is meant to provide an understanding of how varied the causes of proctitis can be and to suggest how the problem can be approached in an orderly fashion, the subject is too complicated for complete coverage in these pages. Each case must be individualized and the discussion pursued with the treating physician.

Epididymitis

In young, sexually active men, epididymitis is usually a complication of sexually acquired urethritis due to gonorrhea or *Chlamydia.* In older men, however, epididymitis is more often caused by nonsexually acquired urinary-tract infections.

The epididymis, a coiled tube that runs along the back of the testis, forms part of the channel that connects the testis to the urethra, allowing sperm to travel from the testicle out through the penis. Infection in the urethra can travel back, against the tide, causing infection in the epididymis.

The symptoms of epididymitis are pain and swelling of the testicle, usually only on one side; urethral discharge; and discomfort on urination. While usually caused by infection, epididymitis can be caused by injury to the testicle. Another condition, testicular torsion, may produce similar symptoms but needs to be distinguished from epididymitis because it requires prompt surgery. In testicular torsion, the blood supply to the testis is cut off. This condition is more often found in boys than in adult men.

The diagnosis of epididymitis is made by physical examination and by looking for bacteria and white blood cells in the urethral discharge or urine. If no bacteria are found, the presumptive cause of infection is *Chlamydia,* which is treated with tetracycline, 500mg four times a day for at least ten days.

In addition to antibiotics, patients with epididymitis need bed rest because the scrotum needs to be elevated for the infection to drain properly. The combination of antibiotics and bed rest should produce improvement within three days; if it doesn't, the patient should see his doctor again. Sexual partners should also be examined and treated for possible infection with gonorrhea or *Chlamydia.*

Prostatitis

Prostatitis, like epididymitis, is frequently a complication of urethritis. The prostate is a gland that sits below the bladder, encircling part of the urethra. The fluid that the prostate secretes flows into the urethra, forming part of the ejaculate.

The symptoms of prostatitis are vague pelvic and low-back pain, difficulty and discomfort urinating, blood in the ejaculate, and pain on ejaculation.

The diagnosis is based on symptoms and a rectal examination. Because the prostate can be felt when a finger is rubbed along the front wall of the rectum, the doctor will be able to tell whether the gland is swollen and painful.

Since prostatitis can be caused by infection in the urethra, the urine and any urethral discharge should be checked for bacteria. Although it hasn't been proved that *Chlamydia* and *U. urealyticum* cause prostatitis, they are suspected of being able to do so. If no bacteria are found, patients should be treated with tetracycline or erythromycin. Sometimes "prostatitis" occurs without infection, a condition whose correct name is "prostatosis." In this case antibiotics won't help. Hot sitz baths may help alleviate symptoms regardless of what has inflamed the prostate.

THE MEDICAL EXAMINATION

WHERE TO GO FOR THE EXAMINATION

There are three basic choices: a private physician, a prepaid group, or an STD clinic.

The major advantage of a private physician is that one has a specific person to turn to. This setup usually provides the maximum feeling of privacy and the most personal medical care. The practice usually reflects one doctor's style—from the aesthetics of the office to the flexibility of arranging appointments. The disadvantages are that most private doctors work on a fee-for-service basis, each visit is billed separately, laboratory tests and referrals to other doctors usually are not included. Depending on physician and laboratory charges, this can be a costly arrangement—especially when multiple visits and tests are necessary, as they so often are for treating STDs.

Prepaid groups have the advantage that doctors' visits and laboratory fees are usually included in the membership fee. If a patient is seen by a doctor who feels that referral to a specialist is warranted, this additional evaluation takes place at no extra cost, since the specialist is part of the group. Another advantage of this setup is that the enrollment fee often includes hospitalization insurance, whereas the person who goes to a private physician must make separate arrangements for hospital coverage. But the disadvantage of a prepaid group practice is that one has less flexibility in choosing one's doctors. This type of medical care can also strike patients as less "personal."

STD clinics can be run either by the local public-health department or by a private group—such as a gay men's organization. Some studies report that gay men were most satisfied with their treatment for STDs when they attended a gay men's clinic. Since these clinics are designed solely to treat STDs they are usually efficient in doing so. Staff members should know the details of diagnosis and treatment, and public-health clinics are equipped to do contact tracing. Although most young men don't have chronic medical problems such as diabetes or high blood pressure, a drawback of STD clinics is that they don't treat a patient for other medical problems—although they can probably refer him to a doctor who will.

In making a choice, one then has to consider the qualities one wants from the physician. One of the first considerations may be whether one would prefer a gay doctor. A good physician is nonjudgmental, whether he or she is straight or gay. But patients may have specific preferences—a doctor who is young, old, male, female, gay, or straight. In large cities, where there are many doctors, it should be possible to find a physician to suit one's preferences. A patient has to feel comfortable discussing his life, including his sexual orientation and sexual practices.

Other factors to consider include the physician's hospital affiliation and medical expertise. To find out where a doctor admits those patients who require hospital care, one need only ask. The patient should then consider whether this hospital is acceptable.

The doctor's expertise is determined not only by training but also by his or her interests. Is the doctor an internist? A urologist? A dermatologist? A general practitioner? These are the most likely specialties of a physician treating STDs. But regardless of the doctor's training, he or she may have acquired a great deal of expertise in a particular field of interest—such as STDs. These are questions that should be asked directly.

Good qualifications aren't necessarily synonymous with being a good doctor. And owing to variability in individual interactions, a successful relationship between one patient and his doctor doesn't guarantee success with another patient and the same doctor. A prospective patient should ask people he knows and trusts for recommendations, and then evaluate the situation for himself.

THE EXAMINATION

There are three parts to an exam: the history, the physical examination, and the laboratory tests. How extensive each part is depends on the patient's problem and on the setting of the exam. A doctor in a busy STD clinic usually can't afford the time that a private physician will allocate for an exam, especially if it is the patient's first visit to the private physician.

The history is often the critical factor in leading a doctor to the correct diagnosis. It begins with the patient's current complaint: Why is he here now? Then the doctor will ask for details about this problem: When did it start? Is it getting better or worse? . . . etc. Delving into the patient's past history, the next series of questions is about prior medical and surgical illnesses: What STDs has the patient had? What operations? Does he have any allergies? In a complete exam, the patient will be asked about his family history—about the illnesses of parents, siblings, grandparents. The reason is that some diseases seem to run in families: Heart disease and diabetes are two examples.

The next part of the history is very important, particularly in trying to understand the health of a young patient who doesn't yet suffer the chronic illnesses associated with aging. *What sort of work does he do?* This provides clues about occupational hazards, levels of stress, and satisfaction from work. *Whom does he live with?* This also provides information about the levels of stress and satisfaction in the patient's life. *How many cigarettes does he smoke, and for how many years?* Since cigarettes cause heart and lung disease, this can serve as an opportunity for encouraging preventive medicine. *What drugs and medications does he use?* Even vitamins should be mentioned, because diarrhea may be the result of too much vitamin C rather than an infection. *How much alcohol does the patient drink?* Alcohol has many effects on the body, depending on the quantity one drinks. *Who is the patient sexually active with—men, women, or both?* This gives a clue about the STDs he is exposed to. *How active is he—how many different partners does he usually have a month—and are these contacts often anonymous?* These answers suggest the patient's level of risk for STDs and also provide guidelines on how frequently he should be screened for syphilis and gonorrhea. *What orifices does he use?* This information will suggest what diseases to look for and where to look for them.

After this, the doctor may run down a list of questions about all the different body systems, such as the digestive and urinary systems, to uncover any information that may have been left out.

The physical exam follows. The thoroughness of this depends on whether it is a first exam and what the setting is. The exam usually begins by checking the blood pressure and pulse, and then proceeds in orderly fashion from head to toe. After the initial visit, or if one goes to an STD clinic, the examination will be focused on the current problem.

A good STD examination includes careful inspection of the skin, genitals, and rectum. For gay men who practice anal-receptive intercourse or have bowel symptoms, the rectal exam should include a digital exam and a procedure known as "anoscopy." With the patient on bended knees and resting on his elbows, a short instrument—the anoscope—is lubricated and inserted into the rectum. This permits visualization of the rectal lining. There are several diseases—such as rectal warts and syphilis—that can't be diagnosed without anoscopy.

The initial laboratory exam for all sexually active gay men should include screening blood tests for syphilis and hepatitis B (so that patients will know whether they are immune, whether they are carriers, or whether they should be vaccinated). The exam should also include screening cultures for gonorrhea (urethral, rectal, and throat cultures).

Additional tests may be needed if the patient has specific symptoms. How often the tests for gonorrhea and syphilis should be repeated depend on one's risk for STDs. This will be discussed in the next section, "How Often to Go."

A word about laboratory tests in general. Some physicians perform many STD tests in their offices, and the cost of these tests is often less than if they were sent to a commercial lab. But laboratories run by private doctors do not have to be licensed by departments of health, whereas commercial and hospital laboratories generally do. Quality control in the private office depends solely on the physician in charge.

HOW OFTEN TO GO

One should go every time symptoms develop. But in addition, sexually active men who are not in exclusive monogamous relationships, should be screened periodically for syphilis and gonorrhea. These are the only diseases for which regular screening is recommended. The following guidelines are suggestions with merit; clinical trials have not been done to prove their scientific validity. How often one should go depends on one's level of risk.

High-risk patients should be screened once a month. The following criteria put one at high risk:

- more than ten different partners a month
- anonymous sexual encounters
- sex that occurs in bathhouses and bookstores

- rarely bathing before or after sex
- frequent use of mind-altering drugs (because this impairs judgment)
- having sex with partners from New York City, Los Angeles, or San Francisco (because the high rate of STDs in these cities make catching an infection more likely)
- anal-receptive intercourse and oral-anal contact (Fist-fornication is a high-risk practice, not from the STD standpoint but because major tears may make a colostomy necessary.)

Men who are at medium risk should be screened once every three months. The following criteria are considered to put one at medium risk:

- three to nine different partners a month
- having the same partner on several occasions; sexual encounters within a small group
- sex that occurs in rest rooms, parks, bars, or motor vehicles
- oral-genital sex
- occasional washing, occasional drug use, and partners from cities other than New York, San Francisco, and Los Angeles

Low-risk men should be screened every six months to one year. The following practices make one low-risk:

- fewer than three different partners a month
- monogamous sex (both partners must be monogamous)
- sex that occurs in private homes
- always washing, rarely using drugs, and partners from small towns

HEALTH RESOURCES: CLINICS, HOT LINES, AND REFERRAL CENTERS

The following facilities offer information that may be helpful to someone concerned about STDs. In some cases they offer diagnosis, treatment, or both. Sometimes they simply provide referrals. Some resources are specifically for gay men; others are for anyone with an STD problem.

The fact that they are listed here is not meant as a medical endorsement. No information is provided about costs, since these can change frequently. Most organizations that issue printed information request contributions.

Further information can be obtained by contacting:

NATIONAL RESOURCES

The National Coalition of Gay Sexually Transmitted Disease Services (NCGSTDS)
P. O. Box 239
Milwaukee, Wisconsin 53201

Issues *Guidelines and Recommendations for Healthful Gay Sexual Activity* and the NCGSTDS newsletter.

The National Gay Health Education Foundation
P. O. Box 834
Linden Hill, New York 11354

Issues a *National Gay Health Directory.*

National Gay Task Force
80 Fifth Avenue, Suite 1601
New York, New York 10011
(800) 221-7044 (hot line)
(212) 807-6016

Homosexual Health Report
Mary Ann Liebert, Inc., Publishers
157 East 85th Street
New York, New York 10028
(212) 289-2300

National VD Hot Line. Telephone (800) 227-8922
Provides phone referrals to local STD treatment centers.

Centers for Disease Control
Center for Prevention Services
Technical Information Services
1600 Clifton Road
Atlanta, Georgia 30333
Issue several books on STDs.

American Association of Physicians for Human Rights
152 Hedge Road
Menlo Park, California 94025
(415) 327-6642

American Foundation for the Prevention of VD, Inc.
527 Madison Avenue, Suite 1415
New York, New York 10022
Issues a booklet about prevention.

Herpes Resource Center
P. O. Box 100
Palo Alto, California 94302
Publishes a quarterly booklet about herpes.

LOCAL SERVICES (by state and city)

Alaska

Anchorage:
STD Clinic of Anchorage
825 L Street, zip 99501
(907) 264-4611

Arizona

Tucson:

Gay Health Project
P.O. Box 2807, zip 85702
(602) 748-7339

California

Berkeley:

Berkeley Gay Men's Health Collective
2339 Durant Avenue, zip 94702
(415) 548-2570

Gay Switchboard and Counseling
(415) 841-6224

Davis:

Davis Gay Task Force
433 Russell Boulevard, zip 95617
(916) 753-2090

Garden Grove:

Gay Community Center of Orange County
12832 Garden Grove Boulevard, Suite H, zip 92643
(714) 534-3261

Los Angeles:

Gay Community Services Center
1213 North Highland Avenue, zip 90038
(213) 464-7400

L.A. Sex Information Hot Line
8405 Beverly Boulevard, zip 90048
(213) 653-2118

Sacramento:

Sacramento Hepatitis B Project
P.O. Box 160486, zip 95816
(916) 453-8995

San Diego:

Gay Center for Social Services
(619) 692-4297

San Diego Physicians for Human Rights
P.O. Box 16242, zip 92116

San Francisco:

Bay Area Physicians for Human Rights
P.O. Box 14546, zip 94114
(415) 673-3189

Haight Ashbury Free Medical Clinic
558 Clayton Street, zip 94117
(415) 431-1714

The Resource Foundation
130 Church Street, zip 94114
(415) 864-0550

KS Research and Education Foundation
470 Castro Street #207
Box 3360, zip 94114
(415) 864-4376

The KS Clinic—U.C.S.F.
c/o 110 East Court
Petaluma, California 94952
(415) 666-1407

Colorado

Denver:

Gay Community Center of Colorado, Inc.
1436 Lafayette Street, zip 80218
(303) 831-6268 or 837-1598

Gay and Lesbian Health Alliance
P.O. Box 6101, zip 80206
(303) 831-6268

Connecticut

New Haven:

Yale Self-Care Network
17 Hillhouse Avenue, zip 06520

District of Columbia

Washington:

Whitman-Walker Gay Men's VD Clinic
2335 18th Street NW, zip 20009
(202) 332-5295

Florida

Key West:

Monroe County Health Department
Public Service Building
Jr. College Road, zip 33040
(305) 294-1021

Georgia

Atlanta:

Physical Health Committee
Atlanta Gay Center
931 Ponce de Leon
NE Atlanta, zip 30306
(404) 876-5372

AIDS-Atlanta
P.O. Box 52785, zip 30305
(404) 872-0600

Illinois

Chicago:

Howard Brown Memorial Clinic
2676 North Halsted Street, zip 60614
(312) 871-5778

Maryland

Baltimore:

Gay Community Center Clinic
241 West Chase Street, zip 21201
(301) 837-2050

Massachusetts

Boston:

Fenway Community Health Center
16 Haviland Street, zip 02115
(617) 267-7573

Mayor's Task Force on AIDS
c/o Brian McNaught
Mayor's Gay Liaison
1 City Hall Square, zip 02201

Michigan

Ann Arbor:

Gay and Lesbian STD Clinic
207 Fletcher Avenue
University Health Services, zip 48109
(313) 763-4186

Detroit:

Palmer Clinic
22750 Woodward Avenue, Suite 309
Ferndale, Michigan 48220
(313) 823-5653

Ypsilanti:

Washtenaw County VD Clinic
555 Towner, zip 48197
(313) 485-2181

Minnesota

Minneapolis:

Lesbian and Gay Community Service Center, Inc.
124 West Lake Street, Suite E, zip 55408
(612) 827-5614

New York

Albany:

Capital District Gay Community Center
332 Hudson Avenue, zip 12210
(518) 462-6136

Buffalo:

Mattachine Gay Hot Line
P.O. Box 155
Ellicott Station, zip 14205
(716) 881-5335

New York:

Chelsea Health Center
303 Ninth Avenue (at 28th Street), zip 10001
(212) 239-1700

Gay Men's Health Project
74 Grove Street, Room 2RW, zip 10014
(212) 691-6969

Gay Men's Health Crisis
Box 274
132 West 24th Street, zip 10011
(212) 685-4952 (hotline)

New York Blood Center Hepatitis Program
310 East 67 Street, zip 10021
(212) 570-3312

St. Mark's Clinic
88 University Place, zip 10003
(212) 691-8282

Stuyvesant Polyclinic
137 Second Avenue, zip 10003
(212) 674-0220

Ohio

Cleveland:

Free Medical Clinic of Greater Cleveland
12201 Euclid Avenue, zip 44106
(216) 721-4010

Oklahoma

Tulsa:

Oklahomans for Human Rights
1932 C South Cheyenne, zip 94119
(918) 583-7323

Oregon

Portland:

NW Fountain
125 NW 20th Place, zip 97209
(503) 248-1990

Pennsylvania

Philadelphia:

Gay Switchboard
(215) 546-7100

Rittenhouse Medical Association
2031 Locust Street, zip 19103
(215) 567-2031

Philadelphia Community Health Alternative
and Philadelphia AIDS Task Force
P.O. Box 7259, zip 19101
(215) 232-8055

Pittsburgh:

Pittsburgh Free Clinic
121 South Highland Avenue, zip 15206
(412) 661-6604

Texas

Houston:

Montrose Clinic
104 Westheimer, zip 77006
(713) 528-5535

Kaposi Sarcoma Committee of Houston
P.O. Box 1155
3317 Montrose, zip 77006
(713) 666-8251

Virginia

Richmond:

Fan Free Clinic
1721 Hanover Avenue, zip 23220
(804) 358-8538

Washington

Seattle:

Seattle Gay Clinic
P.O. Box 20066, zip 98102
(206) 329-8390

Wisconsin

Madison:

Blue Bus Clinic
1552 University Avenue, zip 53706
(608) 262-7440

Milwaukee:

Brady East STD Clinic
1240 East Brady Street, zip 53202
(414) 272-2144

Health Department, Social Hygiene Clinic
841 North Broadway, Room 110, zip 53202
(414) 278-3631

CANADA

Quebec

Montreal:

Montreal Health Press
P.O. Box 1000
Station G, zip H 2 W 2 N 1
(514) 272-5441

THE COSTS OF STD TESTING

STD testing can be expensive, particularly when the tests need to be repeated—as they often do. The prices here do not include the cost of a doctor's visit.

The prices listed below are meant to serve as guidelines for what these tests cost. They are based on the prices charged by a few commercial laboratories.

AMEBAS AND GIARDIA

stool exam	$30

CHLAMYDIA

culture	$55

CYTOMEGALOVIRUS

antibodies in the blood	$40

EPSTEIN-BARR VIRUS

antibodies in the blood	$55

HEPATITIS

(Some labs offer a test that includes several of the markers listed below at a lower cost than if each test is ordered separately.)

hepatitis A antibody (IgM and IgG)	$30
hepatitis B core antibody	$35
hepatitis B surface antibody	$20
hepatitis B surface antigen	$20
hepatitis B *e* antigen and *e* antibody	$50
Liver-function tests. These are the ones that show whether the liver is inflamed. Most of the liver function tests (SGOT, LDH, alkaline phosphatase, and bilirubin) are included in a broader test called a "chemistry screen."	$15

HERPES

herpes type 1 and 2 antibody	$75
herpes culture	$55

HLA TYPING

HLA-DR5 (This is the genetic marker shared by 60 percent of the men with AIDS who have developed Kaposi's sarcoma.)	$95

GONORRHEA

culture (This is the price of culturing one site—throat, urethra, or rectum. Often all three must be cultured. Some labs offer a lower price if all three are done together than if each is done separately.)	$15
Gram stain	$10

SALMONELLA AND SHIGELLA

stool culture (Some labs routinely do a separate culture for *Campylobacter;* most require a separate test.)	$25

SYPHILIS

VDRL blood test (The FTA-ABS—which is the specific test for syphilis—is usually done automatically if the VDRL is positive.)	$10

GENERAL TESTS

(These may be done as part of a routine physical or for specific reasons.)

complete blood count	$10
urinalysis	$7

THE MALE ANATOMY

This is a brief sketch of what the genitourinary system looks like and what each of its components does.

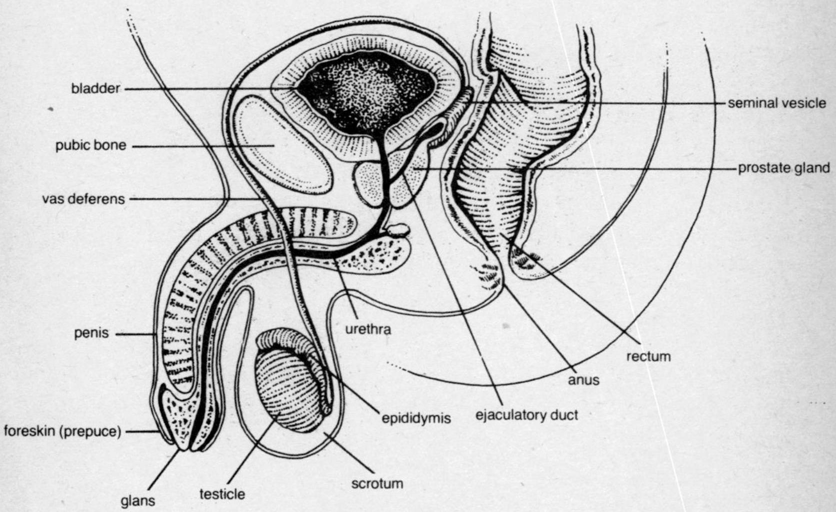

The male sex organs

The Penis

The penis is made up of three cylinders that are erectile tissue. During sexual arousal, blood no longer drains out of these cylinders and the penis becomes erect. The GLANS is the expanded tip of the penis and is actually the end of one of the cylinders, known as the "corpus spongiosum." An extra piece of skin, known as the FORESKIN OR PREPUCE, covers the glans in the uncircumcised male. The opening at the tip of the penis is the urethra, through which urine and semen flow.

The Testes

The testes are the organs that produce sperm and male sex hormones. These hormones cause secondary sexual characteristics such as pubic hair and beard growth.

The Scrotum

The scrotum is a muscular sac that supports the testes. Since sperm function is impaired by high body temperatures, the scrotum—which supports the testes outside the body cavity—is part of the structure that ensures optimum sperm function.

The Urethra

This is a tube-like structure that serves as a conduit for urine and semen. The urethra runs from the BLADDER, where urine is stored, through the entire length of the penis.

The Prostate

The prostate is the largest of several glands secreting fluids that become part of the ejaculate. The prostate sits just below the bladder and encircles the urethra as it exits from the bladder, like a ring around the neck of a funnel. The urethra and prostate can cause problems for each other. If the prostate enlarges, which it does very frequently in older men, it can obstruct urinary outflow through the urethra. If one gets an infection in the urethra, this can spread into the prostate.

The Epididymis

This is the first part of the duct system that transports sperm to the urethra. The epididymis is a structure of about one and a half inches that sits along the back of the testis. (There are two epididymes—one for each testis.) If unwound, the epididymis is approximately 16-feet-long. It stores sperm and secretes a mucoid substance that facilitates its transport.

The Vas Deferens

This is also a duct. It connects the epididymis to the urethra.

The Seminal Vesicles

There are two of these glands, which are sac-like attachments to the vas deferens just before the vas joins the urethra. They contribute a yellowish sticky fluid to the ejaculate.

The Anus

The anus is not part of the genitourinary system, but deserves mention since it features prominently in the discussion of STDs. The anus is the opening of the RECTUM, which is the end of the large bowel, also known as the COLON.

GLOSSARY

abscess: A walled-off collection of pus.

acute: An acute illness is a short-term illness, as opposed to a chronic illness, which is long-term. Acute symptoms are those that start suddenly or that are severe.

AIDS: The acquired immune deficiency syndrome.

anilingus: Oral-anal sex. The same as *rimming.*

antibiotic: A medication to treat an infection. Antibiotics work against bacteria, fungi, and protozoans. Drugs against certain viruses are available but are often called "antivirals."

antibody: A protein made by the immune system to protect the body against infection.

antigen: Any stimulus for making antibodies.

anus: Opening of the rectum.

autoimmune diseases: Diseases caused by the immune system attacking a patient's tissues for unknown reasons.

balanitis: Inflammation of the glans penis.

bacterium: A one-celled microorganism that has a rigid cell wall. The cell wall is responsible for the shape and staining properties of bacteria.

bad blood: Another name for syphilis.

Behçet's syndrome: Recurrent genital and oral ulcers are the major features of this syndrome.

biopsy: A tissue sample taken for diagnostic purposes.

bubo: A very large, swollen lymph node caused by infections such as lymphogranuloma venereum.

carcinogenic: Causing cancer.

carrier: Someone who has an infection without having symptoms from it, but who is contagious.

chancre: The lesion of primary syphilis. A "soft chancre" is the lesion of chancroid.

clap: Slang for gonorrhea.

condylomata acuminata: Venereal warts caused by *Papillomavirus.*

condylomata lata: Lesions of secondary syphilis.

congenital: Existing at birth, such as congenital syphilis.

crabs: Pubic lice.

culture: A test used to identify an infectious agent, which involves growing the organism in some medium.

discharge: Fluid that is secreted, often because of inflammation or infection, such as a rectal or urethral discharge.

dermatologist: A physician who is a skin specialist.

endemic: A disease that is constantly present in a community, usually causing recognizable symptoms only in a few.

enteric: Having to do with the bowel. Enteric bacteria are those that normally live in the gut.

epidemic: A disease which is only occasionally present in a human community. Epidemic diseases tend to be much more severe than endemic ones.

epidemiology: The study of disease patterns. Factors often considered are the age, location, and occupation of persons with the disease.

epididymis: The first part of the tube connecting the testis to the urethra.

epididymitis: Inflammation of the epididymis, causing pain and swelling of the testicle.

fellatio: Oral-penile sex.

fistula: An abnormal passageway between internal organs or between an internal organ and the skin. Usually the result of severe inflammation.

fissure: A superficial tear, as in rectal fissure. This is in contrast to a tear through the full thickness of the rectal wall, which can result from fist-fornication.

fungus: A one-celled fungus is also referred to as a yeast; *Candida* is a yeast. Mushrooms and molds are multicelled fungi.

gland: Often used interchangeably with "lymph node." But "gland" can also refer to an organ that secretes fluid, such as the prostate gland.

Gram stain: A special stain used to characterize bacteria before they are examined under the microscope. Bacteria are either Gram-negative—in which case they look pink—or Gram-positive—in which case they look dark blue.

hemmorhoids: Dilated rectal veins that can bleed and hurt.

hepatitis: Inflammation of the liver, causing jaundice, loss of appetite, and right upper-abdominal pain.

immune system: The body's internal defense system against infection, transplanted organs, and cancer.

incidence: The number of new cases that occur during a set period of time. The total number of cases (which is the prevalence) may be much higher than the incidence of the disease. The incidence of genital herpes is 200,000 to 500,000 per year, but the prevalence is 20 million.

incubation period: The time between exposure to the toxic agent and developing signs and symptoms of the disease.

inflammation: The response of tissues to injury. The injury can be caused by infection or trauma, or it may have no apparent cause.

interferon: A protein made by white blood cells that are infected with a virus to prevent this virus from infecting other cells.

internist: A physician who treats adults for medical (as opposed to surgical) problems.

Jarisch-Herxheimer reaction: Flu-like symptoms that develop when someone with syphilis is treated with antibiotics, resulting from breakup of the bacteria and not from an allergy to the medication.

jaundice: A yellow tint to the skin and eyes due to the buildup of the blood pigment bilirubin. One of the signs of hepatitis.

lesion: A general word that denotes a wound, injury, or pathologic change in tissues. Examples are skin lesions and lesions seen on X-rays.

lymphocyte: A small white blood cell that has a round, dark blue appearance under the microscope and is the basis of the immune system.

lues: An old-fashioned name for syphilis; derived from the Latin, meaning "plague" or "contagious disease."

mucous lining or membrane: The shiny tissue which lines body cavities that are exposed to the outside world, such as the mouth or rectum.

mutagenic: Causing genetic mutation. Mutagenic substances are often suspected of also being carcinogenic.

opportunistic: An opportunistic organism is one that ordinarily doesn't cause disease but may cause severe infections in patients whose immune defenses have been lowered by either disease or medical treatment of disease.

parasite: An organism that is not metabolically self-sufficient and therefore lives off another organism. Protozoans are often referred to as parasites.

pharynx: The medical term for the throat. "Pharyngeal" is the adjective.

proctitis: Inflammation of the rectum, causing rectal pain and discharge.

protozoan: A one-celled animal.

Reiter's syndrome: An illness consisting of arthritis, urethritis, and conjunctivitis whose cause is unknown.

rimming: Oral-anal sex.

RPR (Rapid Plasma Reagin): A screening blood test for syphilis.

STD: The acronym for sexually transmitted disease.

stricture: An abnormal narrowing of tube-like organs such as the rectum or urethra.

syndrome: An illness that has a distinct constellation of features. Many syndromes do not have a known cause.

systemic: Generalized or widespread. A systemic illness contrasts with a localized illness—the flu is a systemic illness, whereas a boil is a localized problem.

titer: The strength of a solution. An antibody titer is a measure of the quantity of the antibody. A high titer means that there is a lot of antibody. Changes in antibody titers can be used to document recovery from an infection and to provide circumstantial evidence about the cause of an illness.

urethra: The tube connecting the bladder to the outside world.

urethritis: Inflammation of the urethra, causing pain and frequency of urination and a penile discharge.

VDRL (Venereal Disease Research Laboratory): A screening blood test for syphilis. The VDRL is also used to measure the response to treatment and to evaluate the possibility of reinfection.

venereal: The word means "sexually related"; it is derived from Venus, the goddess of love.

virus: A virus is the smallest microorganism to cause infections in man. It is technically a parasite because it depends on a living host cell for survival. Viruses contain either DNA or RNA.

BIBLIOGRAPHY

Journal Abbreviations in Bibliography

American Family Physician (*AFP*)
American Journal of Epidemiology (*Am J*)
American Journal of Dermatopathology (*Am J of Dermatopathology*)
American Journal of Medicine (*Am J Med*)
American Journal of Opthalmology (*Am J Opth*)
American Journal of Public Health (*AJPH*)
Annals of Emergency Medicine (*Ann Emerg Med*)
Annals of Internal Medicine (*Ann Int Med*)
Annals of Ophthalmology (*Ann of Ophth*)
Archives of Dermatology (*Arch Dermatol*)
British Journal of Venereal Diseases (*Br J Vener Dis*)
Bulletin of New York Academy of Medicine (*Bull NY Acad Med*)
Canadian Medical Association Journal (*CMA Journal*)
Hospital Practice (*Hosp Prac*)
International Journal of Dermatology (*Int J of Dermatology*)
Johns Hopkins Medical Journal (*Johns Hopkins Med J*)
Journal of the American Medical Association (*JAMA*)
Journal of Clinical Pathology (*J of Clinical Pathology*)
Journal of Homosexuality (*J of Homosexuality*)
Medical Letter (*Med Letter*)
Medical World News (*Med World News*)
Morbidity and Mortality Weekly Report (*MMWR*)
New England Journal of Medicine (*NEJM*)
New York State Medical Journal (*New York State J Med*)
Postgraduate Medicine (*Postgraduate Med*)
Sexually Transmitted Diseases (*Sex Trans Dis*)
Southern Medical Journal (*South Med J*)

GENERAL STD BIBLIOGRAPHY

Centers for Disease Control. *Quality Assurance Guidelines for STD Clinics, 1982.* U.S. Department of Health and Human Services, publication no. 00-4066.

——— STD Fact Sheet (edition 35) U.S. Department of Health and Human Services, publication no. 81-8195.

——— *Sexually Transmitted Disease Statistical Letter, 1980.* U.S. Department of Health and Human Services, publication no. 99-1404.

——— "Sexually Transmitted Diseases Treatment Guidelines 1982." *MMWR,* August 20, 1982.

Isselbacher, Kurt J. et al, eds. *Harrison's Principles of Internal Medicine.* 9th ed. New York: McGraw-Hill, 1980.

National Institutes of Allergy and Infectious Diseases. *Sexually Transmitted Diseases, 1980 Status Report,* NIAID Study Group. NIH publication no. 81-2213.

INTRODUCTION

American Medical Association. "Health Care Needs of a Homosexual Population." *JAMA* 248, no. 6(1982):736–39.

Babb, Richard R. "Sexually Transmitted Infections in Homosexual Men." *Postgraduate Med* 65(1979):215-18.

Bolan, Robert K. "Sexually Transmitted Diseases in Homosexuals: Focusing the Attack" (editorial). *Sex Trans Dis* 8(1981):293–97.

Brandt, Edward N., Jr. "Physicians and Sexually Transmitted Diseases: A Call to Action" (editorial). *JAMA* 248, no. 16(1982):2032.

Darrow, William W. "Social and Psychological Aspects of the Sexually Transmitted Diseases: A Different View."*Cutis* 27(1981):307–20.

Darrow, William W. et al. "The Gay Report on Sexually Transmitted Diseases." *AJPH* 71(1981):1004–11.

Dritz, Selma K. "Medical Aspects of Homosexuality" (editorial) *NEJM* 302(1980):463–64.

Drusin, Lewis M. "The Embarrassing Epidemic" (editorial). *Sex Trans Dis* 9(1982):149–50.

Felman, Yehudi M. et al. "Incidence and Epidemiology of Sexually Transmitted Disease." *Current Therapeutic Research* 26(1979 supp):665–74.

———. "Epidemiological Approach to Control of Sexually Transmitted Disease." *New York State J Med* 79(1979):745–46.

Handsfield, H. Hunter. "Sexually Transmitted Diseases in Homosexual Men" (editorial). *AJPH* 71(1981):989–90.

Holmes, King K. "Future Directions in Research on Sexually Transmitted Diseases in Homosexual Men." *J of Homosexuality* 5(1980):317–24.

Judson, Franklyn N. et al. "Comparative Prevalence Rates of Sexually Transmitted Diseases in Heterosexual and Homosexual Men." *Am J Epid* 112(1980):836–43.

National Institutes of Allergy and Infectious Diseases. *Sexually Transmitted Diseases, 1980 Status Report.* NIAID Study Group. NIH Publication no. 81-2213.

Ostrow, David G. "Factors Adversely Affecting Research in Sexually Transmitted Diseases Among Gay Men." *J of Homosexuality* 5(1980):329–32.

Owen, William F., Jr. "Sexually Transmitted Diseases and Traumatic Problems in Homosexual Men." *Ann Int Med* 92(1980):805–08.

Sandholzer, Terry A. "Physician Attitudes Affecting the Incidence of Sexually Transmitted Diseases in Homosexual Males." *J of Homosexuality* 5(1980):325–27.

Stamm, Walter E. et al. "Clinical Training in Venereology in the United States and Canada." *JAMA* 248, no. 16 (1982):2020–24.

Willcox, R. R. "Sexual Behavior and Sexually Transmitted Disease Patterns in Male Homosexuals." *Br J Vener Dis* 57(1981):167–69.

William, Daniel C. "Sexually Transmitted Diseases in Gay Men: An Insider's View." *Sex Trans Dis* 6(1979):278–80.

THE ACQUIRED IMMUNE DEFICIENCY SYNDROME (AIDS)

"Acquired Immune Deficiency: Health Care Workers at Risk, Too." *Med World News,* Dec. 6, 1982, pp. 8–14.

Bishop, Jerry E. "Lethal New Ailment Claims Another Group of Victims: Children." *Wall Street Journal,* Dec 10, 1982.

Centers for Disease Control. "Epidemiologic Aspects of the Current Outbreak of Kaposi's Sarcoma and Opportunistic Infections." *NEJM* 306(1982):248–52.

———. "Pneumocystis Pneumonia." *MMWR,* June 5, 1981.

———. "Kaposi's Sarcoma and Pneumocystis Pneumonia among Homosexual Men." *MMWR,* July 3, 1981.

———. "Follow-up on Kaposi's Sarcoma and *Pneumocystis* Pneumonia." *MMWR,* Aug. 28, 1981.

———. "Persistent, Generalized Lymphadenopathy Among Homosexual Males." *MMWR,* May 21, 1982.

———. "Diffuse, Undifferentiated Non-Hodgkin's Lymphoma Among Homosexual Males." *MMWR,* June 4, 1982.

———. "Update on Kaposi's Sarcoma and Opportunistic Infections in Previously Healthy Persons." *MMWR,* June 11, 1982.

———. "A Cluster of Kaposi's Sarcoma and *Pneumocystis carinii* Pneumonia among Homosexual Male Residents of Los Angeles and Orange Counties, California." *MMWR,* June 18, 1982.

———. "Opportunistic Infections and Kaposi's Sarcoma Among Haitians in the United States." *MMWR,* July 9, 1982.

———. "*Pneumocystis carinii* Pneumonia Among Persons with Hemophilia A." *MMWR,* July 16, 1982.

———. "Update on Acquired Immune Deficiency Syndrome (AIDS)—United States." *MMWR,* Sept. 24, 1982.

———. "Cryptosporidiosis: Assessment of Chemotherapy of Males with Acquired Immune Deficiency Syndrome (AIDS)." *MMWR,* Nov. 12, 1982.

———. "Update on Acquired Immune Deficiency Syndrome (AIDS) Among Patients with Hemophilia A." *MMWR,* Dec. 10, 1982.

———. "Immunodeficiency among Female Sexual Partners of Males with Acquired Immune Deficiency Syndrome (AIDS)." *MMWR,* Jan. 7, 1983.

———. "Acquired Immune Deficiency Syndrome (AIDS) in Prison Inmates." *MMWR,* Jan. 7, 1983.

Clemmesen, Johannes. "Kaposi Sarcoma in Homosexual Men: Is It a New Disease?" (letter) *Lancet,* July 3, 1982, pp. 51–52.

"CNS Toxoplasmosis Crops up in Patients with AIDS." *Med World News,* Nov. 22, 1982, pp. 24–25.

Colen, B.D.

———. "Epidemic Baffles U.S. Experts." *Newsday,* Sept. 12, 1982.

———. "Sexual Habits a Key to Syndrome." *Newsday,* Sept. 13, 1982.

———. "Mystery Epidemic Is Linked to Haitians." *Newsday,* Sept. 14, 1982.

———. "A Potential Threat to U.S. Blood Supply." *Newsday,* Sept. 15, 1982.

Daling, Janet R. et al. "Correlates of Homosexual Behavior and the Incidence of Anal Cancer." *JAMA* 247(1982):1988–90.

Doll, Donald C. et al. "Burkitt's Lymphoma in a Homosexual." (letter) *Lancet,* May 1, 1982, pp. 1026–27.

Drew, W. Lawrence et al. "Cytomegalovirus and Kaposi's Sarcoma in Young Homosexual Men." *Lancet,* July 17, 1982, pp. 125–27.

"Drugs for Treatment of Systemic Fungal Infections." *Med Letter,* Apr. 2, 1982.

Durack, David T. "Opportunistic Infections and Kaposi's Sarcoma in Homosexual Men." (editorial) *NEJM* 305(1981):1465–67.

Fain, Nathan. "Is Our Lifestyle Hazardous to our Health?" (parts I and II) *The Advocate,* Mar. 18, 1982; Apr. 1, 1982.

Fauci, Anthony S. "The Syndrome of Kaposi's Sarcoma and Opportunistic Infections: An Epidemiologically Restricted Disorder of Immunoregulation." (editorial) *Ann Int Med* 96(1982):777–79.

Festenstein, Freda. "Cytomegalovirus Infection Simulating Lymphoma in a Homosexual Man." (letter) *Lancet,* May 29, 1982, pp. 1248–49.

Follansbee, Stephen E. et al. "An Outbreak of *Pneumocystis carinii* Pneumonia in Homosexual Men." (part I) *Ann Int Med* 96(1982):705–13.

Food and Drug Administration. "Research on AIDS." *FDA Drug Bulletin* 12(1982):21–23.

Friedman-Kien, Alvin E. et al. "Disseminated Kaposi's Sarcoma in Homosexual Men." (part I) *Ann Int Med* 96(1982):693–700.

Gapen, Phyllis. "Neurological Complications Now Characterizing Many AIDS Victims." *JAMA* 248(1982):2941–42.

Goedert, James J. et al. "Amyl Nitrite May Alter T Lymphocytes in Homosexual Men." *Lancet,* Feb. 20, 1982, pp. 412–14.

Gold, Kenneth D. et al. "Aggressive Kaposi's Sarcoma in a Heterosexual Drug Addict." (letter) *NEJM* 307(1982):498.

Gottlieb, Geoffrey J. et al. "A Preliminary Communication on Extensively Disseminated Kaposi's Sarcoma in Young Homosexual Men." *Am J of Dermatopathology* 3(1981):111–14.

Gottlieb, Michael S. et al. "*Pneumocystis Carinii* Pneumonia and Mucosal Candidiasis in Previously Healthy Homosexual Men." *NEJM* 305(1981):1425–30.

Greenberg, Frank et al. "Screening for Risk of Acquired Immune Immune-Deficiency Syndrome." (letter) *NEJM* 307(1982):1521–22.

Groopman, Jerome E. et al. "Kaposi's Sarcoma: Why a 'Homosexual Disease'?" *Hosp Prac,* May 1982, pp. 64 F–T.

Gunby, Phil. "T-cell Stimulator Undergoes Diverse Testing." *JAMA* 248(1982):807.

Holland, Gary N. et al. "Ocular Disorders Associated with a New Severe Acquired Cellular Immune Deficiency Syndrome." *Am J Ophth* 93:393–402.

Hughes, Walter T. "*Pneumocystis Carinii* Pneumonia." *NEJM* 297(1977):1381–83.

———. "*Pneumocystis* Pneumonia: A Plague of the Immunosuppressed." *Johns Hopkins Med J* 143(1978):184–92.

Hymes, Kenneth B. et al. "Kaposi's Sarcoma in Homosexual Men—A Report of Eight Cases." *Lancet,* Sept. 19, 1981, pp. 598–600.

"Immune Deficiency." *Med World News,* Aug. 16, 1982, pp. 7–9.

Jensen, Ole M. et al. "Burkitt's Lymphoma in a Homosexual." *Lancet,* May 1, 1982, pp. 1026–27.

"Ketoconazole." *Med Letter,* Oct. 2, 1981.

Kondlapoodi, P. "Anorectal Cancer and Homosexuality." (letter) *JAMA* 248(1982):2114–15.

Kornfeld, Hardy et al. "T-lymphocyte Subpopulations in Homosexual Men." *NEJM* 307(1982):729–31.

Krick, James A. et al. "Toxoplasmosis in the Adult–An Overview." *NEJM* 298(1978):550–53.

Macek, Catherine. "Acquired Immunodeficiency Syndrome Cause(s) Still Elusive." *JAMA* 248(1982):1423–31.

Marmor, Michael et al. "Risk Factors for Kaposi's Sarcoma in Homosexual Men." *Lancet,* May 15, 1982, pp. 1083–87.

Marx, Jean L. "New Disease Baffles Medical Community." *Science* 217(1982):618–21.

Masur, Henry et al. "An Outbreak of Community-Acquired *Pneumocystis carinii* Pneumonia." *NEJM* 305(1981):1431–36.

Menitove, Jay E. at al. "T-lymphocyte Subpopulations in Patients with Classic Hemophilia Treated with Cryoprecipitate and Lyphilized Concentrates." *NEJM* 308(1983):83–86.

Mildvan, Donna et al. "Opportunistic Infections and Immune Deficiency in Homosexual Men." (part I) *Ann Int Med* 96(1982):700–704.

Miller, James R. et al. "Progressive Multifocal Leukoencephalopathy in a Male Homosexual with T-cell Immune Deficiency." *NEJM* 307(1982):1436–37.

Morris, Lynn et al. "Autoimmune Thrombocytopenic Purpura in Homosexual Men." (part I) *Ann Int Med* 96(1982):714–17.

"New Cases of Kaposi's Sarcoma, AID Found in Heterosexual Men." *Hosp Pract,* Sept. 1982, pp. 48 A–O.

New York City Department of Health. "A.I.D.S.—Surveillance Update." Dec. 22, 1982.

Siegal, Frederick P. et al. "Severe Acquired Immunodeficiency in Male Homosexuals, Manifested by Chronic Perianal Ulcerative Herpes Simplex Lesions." *NEJM* 305(1981):1439–44.

Snider, William D. et al. "Primary Lymphoma of the Nervous System Associated with Acquired Immune-Deficiency Syndrome." (letter) *NEJM* 308(1983):45.

Stahl, Rosalyn E. et al. "Immunologic Abnormalities in Homosexual Men." *Am J Med* 73(1982):171–78.

Thomsen, Henrik K. et al. "Kaposi Sarcoma Among Homosexual Men in Europe." (letter) *Lancet,* Sept. 26, 1981, p. 688.

Urmacher, C. et al. "Outbreak of Kaposi's Sarcoma with Cytomegalovirus Infection in Young Homosexual Men." *Am J Med* 72(1982):569–75.

Walzer, Peter D. "*Pneumocystis carinii* Infection." *South Med J* 70(1977):1330–37.

Whitley, Richard J. et al. "Early Vidarabine Therapy to Control the Complications of Herpes Zoster in Immunosuppressed Patients." *NEJM* 307(1982):971–75.

William, Dan. "If AID Is an Infectious Disease . . ." *New York Native,* Aug. 16–29, 1982.

Williams, George et al. "Cytomegalic Inclusion Disease and *Pneumocystis carinii* Infection in an Adult." *Lancet,* Oct. 29, 1960, pp. 951–55.

Wood, Ronald W. (letter about nitrite inhalants) *NEJM* 306(1982):932–33.

Zakowski, Phillip et al. "Disseminated *Mycobacterium avium-intracellulare* Infection in Homosexual Men Dying of Acquired Immunodeficiency." *JAMA* 248(1982):2980–82.

Ziegler, John L. et al. "Outbreak of Burkitt's-like Lymphoma in Homosexual Men." *Lancet,* Sept. 18, 1982, pp. 631–33.

HEPATITIS

Bolan, Robert K. et al. "Hepatitis B and Sexual Practices." *Ann Int Med* 96(1982):678.

Centers for Disease Control. "Inactivated Hepatitis B Virus Vaccine." *Ann Int Med* 97(1982):379–83.

Centers for Disease Control. "Hepatitis B Virus Vaccine Safety; Report of an Inter-Agency Group." *MMWR* 31, no. 34 (1982).

Dzik, Walter H. et al. "Hepatitis B Viral Infection." (parts I and II) *AFP,* Aug. 1982, pp. 119–26; Sept. 1982, pp. 135–42.

Favero, Martin S. et al. "Guidelines for the Care of Patients Hospitalized with Viral Hepatitis." *Ann Int Med* 91(1979):872–76.

Fawaz, Karim A. et al. "Viral Hepatitis in Homosexual Men." *Gastroenterology* 81(1981):537–38.

Felman, Yehudi M. et al. "Sexually Transmitted Viral Hepatitis." *New York State J Med,* Jan. 1980, pp. 64–66.

Francis, Donald P. et al. "The Report of Hepatitis B with Vaccine—Report of the Centers for Disease Control Multi-Center Efficacy Trial Among Homosexual Men." *Ann Int Med* 97(1982):362–66.

"Hepatitis B." *Sexual Medicine Today,* Aug. 1982, pp. 20–26.

"Hepatitis B Vaccine." *Med Letter,* Aug. 20, 1982.

Krugman, Saul et al. "Viral Hepatitis, Type B." *NEJM* 300(1979):101–106.

Mulley, Albert G. et al. "Indications for the Use of Hepatitis B Vaccine, Based on Cost-Effectiveness Analysis." *NEJM* 307(1982):644–52.

Reiner, Neil E. et al. "Asymptomatic Rectal Mucosa Lesions and Hepatitis B Surface Antigen." *Ann Int Med* 96(1982):170–73.

Schreeder, Marshall T. et al. "Epidemiology of Hepatitis B Infection in Gay Men." *J of Homosexuality* 5, no. 3 (1980):307–10.

Shorey, James. "Sexually Transmitted Hepatitis." *Consultant,* June 1982, pp. 173–81.

Stevens, Cladd E. "Hepatitis B Virus Infection in Homosexual Men." Abstract from American Society for Microbiology Conference, Sept. 8–10, 1982, NYC.

Skinhoj, P. et al. "Chronic Hepatitis B Infection in Male Homosexuals." *J of Clinical Pathology* 32(1979):783–85.

Szmuness, Wolf et al. "Hepatitis B Vaccine. *NEJM* 303(1980):833–41.

———. "Prevalence of Hepatitis B 'e' Antigen and Its Antibody in Various HBsAg Carrier Populations." *Am J of Epidemiology* 113, no. 2:113–21.

Viola, L. A. et al. "Natural History of Liver Disease in Chronic Hepatitis B Surface Antigen Carriers." *Lancet,* Nov. 21, 1981, pp. 1156–59.

GI BLUES

General Articles

Felman, Yehudi M. et al. "Sexually Transmitted Enteric Diseases." *Bull NY Acad Med* 55(1979):533–39.

Heller, Michael. "The Gay Bowel Syndrome: A Common Problem of Homosexual Patients in the Emergency Department." *Ann Emerg Med* 9(1980):487–93.

Silfen, Eric Z. et al. " 'Gay Bowel' Syndrome." *Consultant,* July 1982, pp. 85–94.

William, Daniel C. "Sexually Transmitted Enteric Pathogens in Male Homosexual Population." *New York State J of Med,* Nov. 1977, pp. 2050–52.

William, Daniel C. "Enteric Diseases." *Cutis* 27(1981):278–84.

The Parasites—Amebas and Giardia

"Drugs for Parasitic Infections." *Med Letter,* Jan. 22, 1982.

Felman, Yehudi M. "Amoebiasis and Giardiasis in New York City: A Response." (letter) *Br J Vener Dis* 56(1980):347–48.

———. "Approaches to Sexually Transmitted Amebiasis." *Bull NY Acad Med* 57(1981):201–206.

Istre, Gregory R. et al. "An Outbreak of Amebiasis Spread by Colonic Irrigation at a Chiropractic Clinic." *NEJM* 307(1982):339–42.

Kean, B. H. et al. "Epidemic of Amoebiasis and Giardiasis in a Biased Population." *Br J Vener Dis* 55(1979):375–78.

Keystone, Jay S. et al. "Intestinal Parasitic Infections in Homosexual Men: Prevalence, Symptoms and Factors in Transmission." *CMA Journal* 123(1980):512–14.

Krogstad, Donald J. et al. "Amebiasis." *NEJM* 298(1978):262–65.

Phillips, Steven C. et al. "Sexual Transmission of Enteric Protozoa and Helminths in a Venereal-Disease-Clinic Population." *NEJM* 305(1981):603–606.

Schmerin, Michael J. et al. "Giardiasis: Association with Homosexuality." *Ann Int Med* 88(1978):801–803.

Wolfe, Martin S. "Giardiasis." *NEJM* 298(1978):319–21.

Bacterial Infections

Sazie, Elizabeth S. M. et al. "Rapid Diagnosis of Campylobacter Enteritis." *Ann Int Med* 96(1982):62–63.

HERPES

Altman, Lawrence K. "Is the Alarm over Herpes Excessive?" *New York Times,* November 2, 1982.

Barry, David W. "Topical Acyclovir for Genital Herpes." (letter) *NEJM* 307(1982):1209–10.

Check, William. "The Herpes Hype." *American Health,* Sept./Oct. 1982, p. 90.

Corey, Lawrence et al. "A Trial of Topical Acyclovir in Genital Herpes Simplex Infections." *NEJM* 306(1982):1313–19.

Corey, Lawrence. "The Diagnosis and Treatment of Genital Herpes." *JAMA* 248, no. 9(1982):1041–49.

Crumpacker, Clyde S. et al. "Resistance to Antiviral Drugs of Herpes Simplex Virus Isolated from a Patient Treated with Acyclovir." *NEJM* 306(1982):343–46.

"The Extent of the Genital Herpes Epidemic—And Symptoms to Look For." *Your Patient and Cancer,* July 1982, p. 13.

"Fear of Toilet Seat Herpes Overblown." *Med World News,* June 21, 1982, p. 28.

Felman, Yehudi M. et al. "Herpes Simplex Virus Infections." *New York State J Med,* Feb. 1979, pp. 179–85.

Goldmeier, D. "Proctitis and Herpes Simplex Virus in Homosexual Men." *Br J Vener Dis* 56(1980):111–14.

"Herpes Simplex—Changing Patterns." *Lancet,* Nov. 7, 1981, pp. 1025–26.

Lerner, A. Martin. "Herpes Simplex Virus: Why Treatment Prospects are Brighter." *Modern Medicine,* May 1982, pp. 108–21.

Luby, James. "Therapy in Genital Herpes." (editorial) *NEJM* 306(1982):1356–57.

"Oral Acyclovir Helps Patients with Initial or Recurrent Genital Herpes." *Med World News,* Nov. 8, 1982, pp. 48–50.

Paroski, Paul A., Jr., et al. "Herpes Proctitis." *New York State J Med,* Feb. 1982, pp. 227–29.

Reeves, William C. et al. "Risk of Recurrence after First Episodes of Genital Herpes." *NEJM* 305(1981):315–19.

"Sex and Herpes." *Medical Aspects of Human Sexuality* 16(1982):34C–34L.

"Some Conclusions About Herpes Emerging." *Internal Medicine News,* May 1–14, 1982, p. 16.

Strassburg, Marc A. "Recurrent Genital Herpes: Reinfection or Reactivation?" (letter) *NEJM* 305(1981):1586–87.

Wingerson, Lois. "Did the Press Stir up Panic over Herpes?" *Med World News,* July 19, 1982.

SYPHILIS

Chapel, Thomas A. "The Signs and Symptoms of Secondary Syphilis." *Sex Trans Dis* 7, no. 4(1980):161–64.

Drusin, Lewis M. "Syphilis." Abstract from American Society for Microbiology, Sept 8–10, 1982, NYC.

Felman, Yehudi M. et al. "Syphilis Serology Today." *Archives of Dermatology* 116(1980):84–89.

Felman, Yehudi M. "How Useful are the Serological Tests for Syphilis?" *Int J of Dermatology* 21(1982):79–81.

Felman, Yehudi M. et al. "Primary Syphilis." *Cutis* 29(1982):122–36.

Felman, Yehudi M. et al. "Secondary Syphilis." *Cutis* 29(1982):322–28.

Rudolph, Andrew H. et al. "Syphilis—Diagnosis and Treatment." *Clinical Obstetrics and Gynecology* 18, no. 1(1975):163–81.

GONORRHEA

Ashford, Winston A. et al "Spectinomycin-Resistant Penicillinase-Producing *Neisseria gonorrhoeae." Lancet,* Nov. 7, 1981, pp. 1035–37.

Braff, Erwin H. "Pharyngeal Gonorrhea." (letter) *JAMA* 248, no. 4(1982):427–28.

Centers for Disease Control. "Infections due to Penicillinase-Producing *Neisseria* Gonorrhea—Florida." *MMWR,* May 29, 1981.

Felman, Yehudi M. et al. "Disseminated Gonococcal Infection." *Cutis* 27(1981):140–51.

Felman, Yehudi M. et al. "Spectinomycin in the Treatment of Anal Gonorrhea." *Sex Trans Dis* 5, no. 4(1978):158–59.

Felman, Yehudi M. et al. "Anorectal Gonococcal Infection." *New York State J Med,* Feb. 1980, pp. 231–33.

Handsfield, H. Hunter et al. "Correlation of Auxotype and Penicillin Susceptibility of *Neisseria gonorrhoeae* with Sexual Preference and Clinical Manifestations of Gonorrhea." *Sex Trans Dis,* No. 7 (1980): pp. 1–5.

Holmes, King K. et al. "Disseminated Gonococcal Infection." *Ann Int Med* 74(1971):979–93.

Janda, William M. et al. "Prevalence and Site-Pathogen Studies of *Neisseria meningitidis* and *N. gonorrhoeae* in Homosexual Men." *JAMA* 244, no. 18(1980):2060–64.

Jick, Hershel et al. "Vaginal Spermicides and Gonorrhea." *JAMA* 248, no. 13(1982):1619–21.

Lebedeff, Denis A. et al. "Rectal Gonorrhea in Men: Diagnosis and Treatment." *Ann Int Med* 92(1980):463–66.

Riccardi, Nicholas B. et al "Laboratory Diagnosis in the Problem of Sus-

pected Gonococcal Infection." *JAMA* 242, no. 24(1979):2703–2705.
Salit, Irving E. et al. "Seroepidemiological Aspects of *Neisseria meningitidis* in Homosexual Men." *CMA Journal,* 126(1982):38–41.
Thatcher, Richard W. "Treatment of Acute Gonococcal Conjunctivitis." *Ann of Ophth,* April 1978, pp. 445–49.
Tice, Andrew W. "Pharyngeal Gonorrhea." *JAMA* 246, no. 23(1981):2717–19.
"Treatment of Sexually Transmitted Diseases." *Med Letter,* Mar. 19, 1982.
William, Daniel C. et al. *"Neisseria meningitidis." JAMA* 242, no. 15(1979):1653–54.
William, Daniel C. et al. "Pharyngeal Carriage of *Neisseria meningitidis* and Anogenital Gonorrhea." *Sex Trans Dis* 7, no. 4(1980):175–77.

THE MINOR STDs

Felman, Yehudi M. et al. "Chancroid." *Cutis* 26(1980):464–78.
Felman, Yehudi M. et al. "Condylomata Acuminata." *New York State J Med,* Oct. 1979, pp. 1747–49.
Felman, Yehudi M. et al. "Genital Molluscum Contagiosum." *Cutis* 26(1980):28–32.
Felman, Yehudi M. et al. "Granuloma Inguinale." *Cutis* 27(1981):364–77.
Felman, Yehudi M. et al. "Lymphogranuloma Venereum." *Cutis* 25(1980):264–310.
Felman, Yehudi M. "Lymphogranuloma Venereum," from *Current Dermatologic Therapy.* Philadelphia: W.B. Saunders Co., 1982.
Felman, Yehudi M. et al. "Pediculosis Pubis." *Cutis* 5(1980):482–90.
Felman, Yehudi M. et al. "Scabies." *Cutis* 25(1980):32–42.
Kampmeier, Rudolph H. "The Establishment of Lymphogranuloma Inguinale (Lymphopathia Venereum) as a Sexually Transmitted Disease." *Sex Trans Dis* 9(1982):146–48.
"Local Outbreak of Chancroid Alarms CDC." *Medical World News,* June 7, 1982, p. 90.
Oriel, J. David. "Genital Warts." *Sex Trans Dis* 8(supp.) (1981):326–29.
Schachter, Julius. "Confirmatory Serodiagnosis of Lymphogranuloma Venereum Proctitis May Yield False-Positive Results Due to Other Chlamydial Infections of the Rectum." *Sex Trans Dis* 8(1981):26–28.

THE "ITISES"

Berger, Richard E. "Acute Epididymitis." (editorial) *Sex Trans Dis* 8(1982):286–88.

Berger, Richard E. et al. "*Chlamydia trachomatis* as a Cause of Acute 'Idiopathic' Epididymitis." *NEJM* 298(1978):301–304.

Felman, Yehudi M. et al. "Nongonococcal Urethritis." *JAMA* 245(1981):381–86.

Holmes, King K. et al. "Etiology of Nongonococcal Urethritis." *NEJM* 292(1975):1199–1205.

Kinghorn, G. R. "Postgonococcal Urethritis." *Br J Vener Dis* 54(1978):112–14.

Quinn, Thomas C. et al. "*Chlamydia trachomatis* Proctitis." *NEJM* 305(1981):195–200.

Quinn, Thomas C. et al. "The Etiology of Anorectal Infections in Homosexual Men." *Am J Med* 71(1981):395–406.

Schachter, Julius. "Chamydial Infections." (three-part series) *NEJM* 298(1978):428–34;298:490–95;298:540–48.

THE MEDICAL EXAMINATION

Bolan, Robert K. "Sexually Transmitted Diseases in Homosexuals: Focusing the Attack." (editorial) *Sex Trans Dis* 8(1981):293–97.

Felman, Yehudi M. et al. "Examining the Homosexual Male for Sexually Transmitted Diseases." *JAMA* 238(1977):2046–47.

Felman, Yehudi M. et al. "Obtaining History of Patient's Sexual Activities." *New York State J. Med,* Nov. 1979, pp. 1879–81.

National Coalition of Gay Sexually Transmitted Disease Services. *Guidelines and Recommendations for Healthful Gay Sexual Activity*. Milwaukee, WI 1982.

Index